Benyamin Chetkow-Yanoov, DSW

Social Work Practice
A Systems Approach
Second Edition

Pre-publication
REVIEWS,
COMMENTARIES,
EVALUATIONS . . .

"*Social Work Practice: A Systems Approach* continues to be an outstanding systems text. In this edition, Dr. Chetkow-Yanoov has fine-tuned his original work to provide more coherence in the organization of content. Some sections contain updated information or reformation of ideas. Subject areas are also easier to locate. A discussion of change versus progress has enhanced this edition. It challenges the reader to consider values and perceptions related to change. The inclusion of additional figures helps the visual learner perceive concepts more clearly. The bibliography has been updated and extended to include the latest information on systems theory.

This book is an essential text for courses in systems theory or as a supplemental text in practice courses at the BSW, MSW, or PhD levels."

Judith Davenport, PhD, LCSW
Director, School of Social Work,
University of Missouri,
Columbia, MO

"In this relatively short and easy-to-read book, Dr. Chetkow-Yanoov manages to introduce the complex world of social work practice in a smooth, systematic, and crystalized manner. The book will be of great value both to beginner students and those interested in understanding what social work practice is all about. This second edition is highly recommended as a primary text for any and all introduction to social work courses."

Ram A. Cnaan, PhD
Associate Professor,
School of Social Work,
University of Pennsylvania

"This book provides a comprehensive review of 'systems approach' and its application to the major domains of social work practice, including administration, management, supervision, individual and group work, and social service intervention, as well as community organization and development. The 'systems approach' is one paradigm that has withstood the test of time in terms of contributing to an understanding of human behaviors and events that often necessitate intervention.

Professor Chetkow-Yanoov has skillfully combined key theoretical and practical elements of 'systems approach' to provide a meaningful and worthwhile book that brings viewpoints and methodologies to bear on the topic of improved methods of human intervention. This work brings into focus the significant elements of social work practice and social service provision across the boundaries of multiple settings. What Chetkow-Yanoov has done with the body of knowledge regarding 'systems approach' is to advocate, in a clear and concise manner, the development of a coherent framework based on a body of ideas, research findings, and practice principles that may be used to guide instructors, students, practitioners, trainers, community developers, managers, supervisors, and others through human services planning, organization, and provision.

Overall, *Social Work Practice: A Systems Approach, Second Edition* is worthy of adaptation as a principal book for social work clinical, management, and community development instruction."

Richard Isralowitz, PhD
Professor and Director,
Graduate Studies Program,
Spitzer Department of Social Work,
Ben Gurion University,
Beer Sheba, Israel

"**D**r. Chetkow-Yanoov has once again made an important contribution to the professional literature in his second edition of *Social Work Practice: A Systems Approach*. Written from the understanding and sympathetic viewpoint of the practitioner, the book is particularly useful. This is reflected in the style of presentation, the frequent use of practice content, and the persuasive stress on applicability. The material belies the perception that systems theory, while rich in concepts, is deficit in application. In true systems style, Chetkow-Yanoov shows how this theory and the models of practice it generates cut across many of the imagined boundaries within the profession and between professions. In particular, he demonstrates the artificiality of macro-micro boundaries that have divided the profession to the detriment of the clients we serve.

This is an excellent example of how theory and practice are inextricably intertwined and how, when the perceptions of a skilled teacher and experienced clinician are combined in one person, concepts emerge that are of considerable assistance to practitioners in enabling them to enrich practice by a sensitive application of such theory."

Francis J. Turner, DSW
Professor Emeritus,
Faculty of Social Work,
Wilfrid Laurier University,
Waterloo, Ontario

The Haworth Press, Inc.

Social Work Practice
A Systems Approach

Second Edition

HAWORTH Social Work Practice
Carlton E. Munson, DSW, Senior Editor

New, Recent, and Forthcoming Titles:

Gerontological Social Work Supervision by Ann Burack-Weiss and Frances Coyle Brennan

Group Work: Skills and Strategies for Effective Interventions by Sondra Brandler and Camille P. Roman

If a Partner Has AIDS: Guide to Clinical Intervention for Relationships in Crisis by R. Dennis Shelby

Social Work Practice: A Systems Approach by Benyamin Chetkow-Yanoov

Elements of the Helping Process: A Guide for Clinicians by Raymond Fox

Clinical Social Work Supervision, Second Edition by Carlton E. Munson

Intervention Research: Design and Development for the Human Services edited by Jack Rothman and Edwin J. Thomas

Forensic Social Work: Legal Aspects of Professional Practice by Robert L. Barker and Douglas M. Branson

Now Dare Everything: Tales of HIV-Related Psychotherapy by Steven F. Dansky

The Black Elderly: Satisfaction and Quality of Later Life by Marguerite M. Coke and James A. Twaite

Building on Women's Strengths: A Social Work Agenda for the Twenty-First Century by Liane V. Davis

Family Beyond Family: The Surrogate Parent in Schools and Other Community Agencies by Sanford Weinstein

The Cross-Cultural Practice of Clinical Case Management in Mental Health edited by Peter Manoleas

Environmental Practice in the Human Services: Integration of Micro and Macro Roles, Skills, and Contexts by Bernard Neugeboren

Basic Social Policy and Planning: Strategies and Practice Methods by Hobart A. Burch

Fundamentals of Cognitive-Behavior Therapy: From Both Sides of the Desk by Bill Borcherdt

Social Work Intervention in an Economic Crisis: The River Communities Project by Martha Baum and Pamela Twiss

The Relational Systems Model for Family Therapy: Living in the Four Realities by Donald R. Bardill

Feminist Theories and Social Work: Approaches and Applications by Christine Flynn Saulnier

Social Work Approaches to Conflict Resolution: Making Fighting Obsolete by Benyamin Chetkow-Yanoov

Principles of Social Work Practice: A Generic Practice Approach by Molly R. Hancock

Nobody's Children: Orphans of the HIV Epidemic by Steven F. Dansky

Social Work in Health Settings: Practice in Context, Second Edition by Toba Schwaber Kerson and Associates

Critical Social Welfare Issues: Tools for Social Work and Health Care Professionals edited by Arthur J. Katz, Abraham Lurie, and Carlos Vidal

Social Work Practice: A Systems Approach, Second Edition by Benyamin Chetkow-Yanoov

Social Work Practice
A Systems Approach

Second Edition

Benyamin Chetkow-Yanoov, DSW

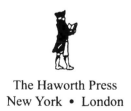

The Haworth Press
New York • London

The Haworth Press, Inc., 10 Alice Street, Binghamton, NY 13904-1580

Cover design by Monica L. Seifert.

Library of Congress Cataloging-in-Publication Data

Chetkow-Yanoov, Benyamin.
   Social work practice : a systems approach / Benyamin Chetkow-Yanoov.–2nd ed.
     p.   cm.
   Includes bibliographical references and index.
   ISBN 0-7890-0246-9 (alk. paper).
    1. Social service. 2. Social systems. 3. Social analysis. I. Title.
HV41.C443 1997
361.3′2–dc21   97-20082
                                                            CIP

CONTENTS

ABOUT THE AUTHOR

Benyamin Chetkow-Yanoov, DSW, is Professor of Social Work at Bar-Ilan University in Israel. While he has consulted and taught primarily in Canada, the United States, and Israel, he has also conducted workshops in Australia, England, Namibia, South Africa, Thailand, and Sweden. He pioneered a master's level course in conflict resolution at Bar-Ilan University's School of Social Work, and has organized training programs for Israelis wanting to learn conflict resolution skills. He is the author of *Social Work Approaches to Conflict Resolution* and has assumed leadership roles in several national organizations for promoting peace and diplomacy. These include *Partnership*, a voluntary association for creating cooperation between Israeli Arabs and Jews, and serving as a consultant for Israel's Ministry of Education. His professional interests include the dynamics of program implementation, community theater, systems analysis, voluntarism, leadership among aging professionals, and community social workers vis-à-vis municipal politicians.

Foreword

The systems model, like all models, serves as a way of looking at an event or phenomenon and providing an orientation for understanding it. The value of a model is not based on its ability to describe a phenomenon or to explain/predict all aspects of its functioning, but rather in its helping us focus on certain aspects of the reality in question. A model helps us analyze events by means of concepts–providing perspective for understanding a specific reality. Like a map, it identifies a system's interdependent components and shows the ongoing relationships among them.

Among systems theoreticians, three basic foci are popular.

- The *atomistic approach* focuses on the individuals as a system, including its components, structure, functions, and history. This approach is usually the basis of social casework or micro intervention.
- The *holistic approach* defines a social system more widely. It is seen as composed of many individual human beings. Now each person is a component or sub-system in the larger system. Structurally and organizationally, the defined system is distinct from its environment (a much larger system). This is the basis for social change or macro intervention efforts.
- The *integrative approach* wrestles with the complexity of being both a whole system for one's components and the component of a larger system simultaneously. In fact, the wholeness of any system, regardless of size or form, is more than a sum of its components. A system has unique characteristics, differentiating it from other systems.

The author of this book speaks from an integrative point of view. The P. family example illustrates this approach clearly. This family is a complete unit, has a unique structure and functioning, and is composed of many sub-units (individual members of the P. family). At the same time, the family is itself a sub-unit within the community system or the environment in which the family resides. Professionally, we have to decide on our intervention focus—each unit (whether the individual, the family, or the community) offering us different opportunities to understand, to diagnose, to set action priorities, and to choose appropriate interventions. Clearly, systems analysis allows us to appreciate the multidimensional complexity of our world.

All systems are characterized by a dynamic balance between stability-conservation and tension-pressure. The former guarantee continuity and identity. The latter create openness, change, and growth, as well as the ability to adjust to internal or external demands. We must reckon the cost/benefits involved in maintaining the system's basic functions and/or in its responding to external pressures. A system whose needs are not met often creates deliberate or unintended pressure for change in its external system (or environment). Of course, an external agent can serve as a catalyst for change among its subsystems.

This book shows us the specific usefulness of a systems approach to professional social work thinking and practice. It contains a rich theoretical basis—explaining basic concepts and emphasizing the interconnections between them. Today, social workers are convinced that the scientific method must be at the basis of their professional training, and knowing a range of theories is essential for effective professional practice. In fact, a constant flow between concrete situations and relevant theories or models has become the essence of sound professional practice.

The systems model is not new. It originated in the natural sciences, and was later adopted by the social-behavioral sciences as well as the mental health field. The wide-ranging presentation of systems in this book is a new operationalization of a known approach. It makes clear that the model can be used both at the micro and macro levels of professional intervention—offering a broad range of practice examples that derive from systems concepts and that help to clarify the concepts. The approach proves relevant to a full kaleidoscope of practice situations, including conflict resolution. With each turn of the kaleidoscope, we see interesting new pictures, examples, recommended exercises, or insights.

The author's conception of systems is compatible with the focal concerns of social workers. It helps us understand human beings in relationship to their social and physical environments. We have a tool to relate to the needs of the individual, group, community, and higher order systems. Living as we do in a complex, dynamic, and changing society, our profession must also develop, become renewed, and adopt up-to-date practice approaches. Moreover, the profession must define and redefine the boundaries of its practice interventions—how much to stay at the micro level and help clients adjust to their social realities, or also to intervene at the macro level and try to bring about wide environmental change.

This question has been at the center of professional discussions for many years. Early this century, social workers chose to confine themselves to a psychiatric form of casework. Activities with larger systems and the search for resources were seen as "less professional." Toward the end of the 1950s, social workers started showing a willingness to become involved in bringing about change in political and economic systems. The author of this book believes that the systems model gives us tools for understanding, analyzing, and intervening with all levels of micro and macro targets. He claims that the systems approach increases our professional sensitivity, and enables us to develop new practice models.

With regard to larger systems (e.g., those at the national and international levels), I feel that systems theory does help us to understand their structures and activities. However, practice realities suggest that the ability of social workers to intervene with such large and complex systems is very limited. To intervene with such targets, we have to utilize rules and ideas from politics, economics, public administration, and the like—"game rules" very different than those used by most professional social workers. Of course, this contention requires empirical verification.

In any case, we still find plenty of tension between adherents of the clinical approach and the social changers. If we want to relate to a wide range of poverty and suffering, we will have to work with many types of social systems. For that, we will have to rely on various bodies of knowledge, and be skilled in a variety of intervention technologies.

Issues of professional competence will continue to concern us. Without doubt, all programs of social work study and training will have to include theoretical and operational content from social systems—along with content from other areas. This book makes a contribution to preparing social workers to be such flexible and creative professionals.

Dr. Shulamith Albeck
School of Social Work
Bar-Ilan University

Acknowledgements

Many people helped me write this book. Years ago, Dr. Francis Turner, then of the Faculty of Social Work at Wilfrid Laurier University (Waterloo, Ontario, Canada), challenged me to expand a short article into a book-length systems analysis of the profession. Dr. Elliott Marcus of the School of Social Work at Bar-Ilan University (Ramat-Gan, Israel) and Ross McClelland of the School of Social Work at UBC (Vancouver, Canada) and David Shewchuk of the Faculty of Social Work at Toronto University helped me overcome my practitioner's resistance to using word processors—and took the drudgery out of writing for me.

Howard Wager, Joseph Katan, Almand Lauffer, Frank Loewenberg, Reuben Schindler, and Allan York each reviewed this text in various stages of its evolution. Their scholarly suggestions and friendly encouragement sustained me at crucial times. Positive classroom feedback from diverse cohorts of students taught me to clarify concepts and to illustrate them through concrete practice examples. Many of these sessions were very exciting and productive for me.

I was blessed by the continuing help and support of my colleague-partner-wife, Bracha. She read every draft critically, pushed me to improve the text repeatedly, and supplied one of the case histories. Her presence has been vital throughout this project.

I learned wisdom from all these wonderful teachers, and I thank them for helping make this book possible.

Introduction

WHY BOTHER WITH SYSTEMS?

This book advocates a systems model of social work, and does so for the following reasons:

1. The systems model enables you to pull together much of what you have found useful in many current models of social work practice (see Chapter 5). In fact, a systems approach should help increase the sensitivity of your practice because systems can: (1) augment other models of practice, and (2) give you tools for linking micro and macro modes of intervention.
2. The systems model is particularly useful for understanding how social workers could sharpen their practice of conflict resolution (see Chapter 6).
3. The systems model should prove useful to students of social environments and of environmental impacts on human growth and behavior (see Chapter 1). It constitutes the basis for ecological models currently popular in the literature of social work.
4. When used correctly (see Chapter 6), the systems model can be used to understand social change and to plan programs of deliberate change.
5. The universality of systems-derived relationships (defined in Chapters 2 and 3) makes this model appropriate for colleagues interested in international social work. Systems analysis should hold true regardless of the cultural or societal setting in which it is practiced.
6. Social workers, like members of other helping professions, can focus on preventing (as well as alleviating) problem conditions if they use systems analysis.

In most problem-solving interventions, practitioners tend to rely on their own unique combination of theoretical knowledge and professional experience. However, choice of intervention strategies is also influenced by your image of what the world is like as well as by the way you think the world functions (e.g., the profession's reliance on such models as psychoanalysis, gestalt, functionalism, ego psychology, task centeredness, existentialism, transactional psychology, or behavior modification). Finally, your choice of action strategies also depends on what is supported by the agency in which you work today, and on the paradigm of the world that is accepted during a particular period of history in a particular society (this idea is elaborated on in Appendix A).

If you become persuaded to adopt a systems orientation in your professional practice, you will look at the world as an organized complexity to be understood as a *whole* in order to grasp it accurately and be able to intervene in it effectively.

CHAPTER OUTLINE

Upon completing your study of this book, you should understand how the systems model can serve as a tool for social work and other helping professions (Greer 1969). You will learn a number of systems concepts and apply what you have learned.

Chapter 1 introduces the term *system* and begins by analyzing a human being as a system. Further analysis focuses on how environments and persons impinge on each other, and on the possibility that components of every environment can be the object of professional intervention. After you have explored this system-environments model, you concentrate on a single human being as a system. You also look at the family, a (person's) participatory environment, the community, the nation, international organizations, and the cosmos—both as environments and as systems. Two exercises are included to help you become familiar with this approach. The chapter closes with a look at ecological theory and some of its implications for social work practice.

Chapter 2 first outlines a systems-oriented model of social work practice and then invites you to look at a record of casework done with a multiproblem family. In order to be able to analyze this case in detail, you are introduced to such systems concepts as boundary (and ecomapping), open and closed systems, vertical and horizontal interactions, feedback, and linkage.

Chapter 3 opens with another problem situation as a way of introducing additional systems concepts such as equilibrium or steady state, input-throughput-output, input overload, manifest and latent functions, functional/dysfunctional, the cycle of system-environment communication, and system coherence. You look again at some of the environments mentioned in Chapter 1, and glance at the implications of relying on a systems model for social work practice.

Chapter 4 emphasizes how systems analysis can lead to a dynamic view of reality. After defining the idea of change, you look at a number of factors that lead to change. Change is analyzed in such systemic terms as inputs-outputs, feedback, boundaries, intersystemic linkages, functions, and external environment. Two case examples are presented: the first, on the personal level, deals with loss and grief; the second, on the organizational level, describes a process of deliberate change in a community center and is analyzed in both traditional and systemic ways.

Chapter 5 focuses on various aspects of social work practice by applying the technology of systems analysis. Needs and problems are defined in systemic terms, and the model is used to analyze client, target, and action subsystems of a case example. After identifying the five systemic stages of an activity or project, you examine a range of appropriate intervention roles. The topic is illustrated with a case example. You study how social work intervention can occur at such points as input (or the boundary), throughput, and feedback—as well as at diverse systemic levels. An Israeli example of efforts to influence social policy is described in systemic terms.

Chapter 6 looks at social work as a profession concerned with conflict resolution in many types of systems. Four components are suggested as basic to all ongoing conflicts, while various combinations of components explain a range of outcomes from cooperation to clashes. In accordance with the above model, you explore a number of ways to de-escalate conflicts and resolve them. The chapter concludes with some comments on conflict mediation as a professional role.

Chapter 7 reviews the systems paradigm used in this book, stressing its usefulness to social workers as well as to other helping professionals. A conflict-filled case history is used to review the major systemic concepts used in the book. The limitations of the systems approach are discussed.

Two appendixes bring this book to a close. The first looks at systems analysis as a model/paradigm. Attention is given to the major paradigm shift (from reductionism to wholeness) that took place in twentieth-century scholarly thinking. Appendix A goes on to describe the appearance of systems-oriented concepts in the literature of both the social sciences and social work. Appendix B outlines an MA level, one-semester course in systems analysis, suggesting relevant content areas for each lesson from various parts of this book.

Throughout the book, diagrams, charts, tables, and exercises are provided in order to help you explore the above topics and develop a holistic approach in your professional practice.

A PERSONAL NOTE

I can remember my own excitement, during my doctoral studies at Brandeis University, when I discovered the systems outlook of Lewin, Merton, Loomis, Parsons, and Warren. Such a linking of social science ideas with my growing practice skills proved a joyful growth experience for me (Chetkow 1963). It expanded my capacity to understand my work world, and made a widened range of options available for helping individuals, organizations, and communities. Since then, my insight into the utility of the model has been expanded by many additional social scientists and practitioners.

I hope this book communicates some of my joy and excitement to you, and that you find this approach helpful in your work.

Benyamin Chetkow-Yanoov
Ramat-Gan, Israel

Chapter 1

Social Systems
and Their Environments

INTRODUCTION TO THE SYSTEMS IDEA

The term *system* is of Greek origin. The word itself is a combination of *syn* (together) and *histanai* (to set). Systems analysts such as J. G. Miller (1955, 1978) claim that things or events, at all levels of complexity, can be viewed as wholes—that a common analytical model can be used to describe the human body, a person, a family, a group, an organization, a neighborhood, a community, a region, a country, an international arrangement (like the European Union, NATO), earth, our solar system, even the universe. As Olsen wrote in 1968:

> A social system is a model of a social organization that possesses a distinct total unity beyond its component parts, that is distinguished from its environment by a clearly defined boundary, and whose subunits are at least partially interrelated within relatively stable patterns of social order. Put even more simply, a social system is a bounded set of interrelated activities that together constitute a single social entity.

A system implies an entity whose parts are seen to make up an orderly and complex totality in accordance with some underlying set of rules. However, this orderliness is the product of the analyst's mind rather than an empirical fact. Warren (1963) summarizes that a system is defined as the relationships among units "which endure through time" and engage in roles "within an enduring pattern of interactions." To put the matter humorously, a systems outlook tends to makes a "mesh" out of everything.

Of course, this book focuses on *human* social systems and on their implications for the people-helping professions. Eventually, you should be able to use systems analysis to describe a diversity of social processes or interactions that happen regularly in specific parts of your workload. Since human beings interact and grow within a variety of surrounding environments, a systems-derived person-environments model seems appropriate for social work intervention. This will become clear as you examine some of the ways in which people interact with their family environments; non-kin environments; and community, national, and regional or international environments.

PEOPLE AS THE FOCUS

Social work scholars like Coulton (1981), Engel (1980), or Germain (1973) emphasize that the object of professional intervention can be a single person, a social collectivity (such as the Red Cross organization), or a wide-ranging environment (such as a metropolitan region or a rain forest). In short, social system analysts perceive their model as equally applicable to the smallest micro and the broadest macro social units.

This chapter focuses on the relationships between individual persons (as systems) and the complex external world (often other systems) which make up the environment. Furthermore, you will note that people are not only the product of their environment but, through interacting with it, are also capable of influencing or changing their external settings.

THE INDIVIDUAL AS A SYSTEM

Every human being is an "organized complexity" worthy of systems analysis. Within the skin of the biological body, the system includes at least the skeletal, assimilatory, respiratory, eliminatory, endocrine, emotional, and nervous subsystems (i.e., components) — all in dynamic interaction. Within this body (an "open" system, which is defined in the next chapter), information is communicated by means of the genes, the senses, electrical impulses, intuition, etc., and many simultaneous feedback channels. Psychosomatic medicine recognizes many cross-boundary interactions between the body's physical-emotional condition and real or imagined threats within its physical-social environments.

Any analysis of an individual person as a system must also take into account what lies beyond that person's boundary. Moos (1976) speaks for many ecologists when he defines environment as including geography, historical perspectives, society, culture, organizations, architecture, weather, noise levels, and even utopian thought. Natural, social, and constructed things or events in the environment can be stressful, inhibiting, challenging, or freeing for specific individuals. Moos's emphasis on human free will rather than on deterministic external forces is refreshing. For the purposes of this book, a multienvironmental model is favored and is elaborated below.

The human body takes in energy (food) from its environment and converts it into cells, tissues, organs, and other matter for self-repairs. All these dynamics mirror a steady-state or growth condition, with continuous inputs contributing to a person's well-being and to other person-systems in the environment. Nonbiological elements such as dreams, thought, memory, willpower, and consciousness contribute to the coherence of this remarkable life form. In an environment that is neither barren nor polluted, a baby will grow from infancy to maturity, from dependency to self-fulfillment, and from relative simplicity to increasing complexity.

A PERSON-ENVIRONMENT MODEL

It is impossible to describe the full complexity of person-environment interactions without resorting to some kind of systems model. As mentioned above, all human beings find themselves within a multiplicity of nearby and distant environments. The following six-layer model is based on the work of Baker (1975), Capelle (1979), Engel (1980), Gotteschalk (1975), and Hall (1966) and is proposed as relevant to everyone. Potentially, all persons interact with elements of the following environments:

1. A nuclear family or multigenerational tribe/clan
2. A participatory environment or reference group

3. A local or municipal community
4. A culture, society, or nation
5. The international scene
6. The cosmos

In any systems analysis, each of these six environments can also be examined as a system, and they all influence, and/or are influenced by, the others. In fact, social workers often have to help their clients deal with the consequences of changes which have taken place in near or distant environments.

The multienvironment model is shown in Figure 1.1. Normal human beings have close family ties (Circle I), and are nurtured by this primary environment. They also participate personally in a range of local (or local branches of) social collectivities such as villages, neighborhoods, schools, factories, recreation centers, stores, health clinics, banks, etc. Even if people are not involved personally with one of these units, awareness of its importance gives them a feeling of belonging (Circle II). In both circles, people experience important primary relationships (e.g., with peers/friends during the first years of life). The importance of job-related friendships, for example, is not sufficiently appreciated by societies when making universal policies for retirement or fighting inflation through enforced disemployment.

Some components of the community environment (Circle III) also lend themselves to primary relationships, but these tend to favor elitist people. If you are a member of the local establishment, you are likely to know the mayor, be a patron of the museum, serve on the executive board of a political party, be invited to join civic agency boards, or act as one of the decision makers in the chamber of commerce. Many studies show that if you are a member of the impoverished lower class, your community involvements may well be much more limited.

The national and international environments (Circles IV and VI), although often the locus of important policy decisions regarding social service standards, are both remote for the average citizen. However, young adults in many parts of the world are finding that one of the serious tension-causing realities of today is the decreasing match between ethnic-cultural-linguistic identity ("people-

FIGURE 1.1. The Six Environments

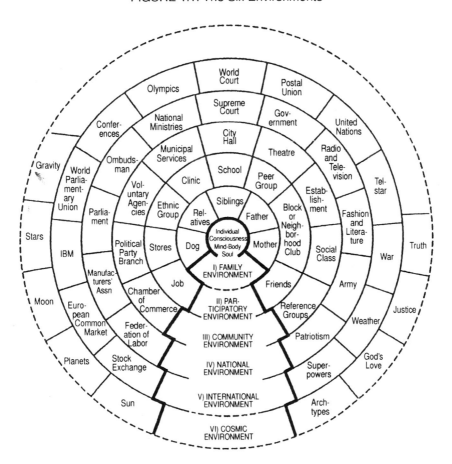

hood") and legal-political-national boundaries ("country"). At the other end, multinational corporations are making national boundaries obsolete.

A common result of feeling cut off from your roots is to identify with a political ideology, become a devotee of some cult, join a hippie commune, engage in fanatic antiestablishment violence, make demands for territorial independence, give fundamentalistic support to some new school or technique of healing, or scapegoat others. Although they appear to be negative, these activities actually help to build a feeling of participation among otherwise disconnected individuals, and seem much less painful (to each of them) than suffering anomie (Fromm 1941).

If your ethnic group is among the stigmatized minorities, national and international issues tend to assume low priority while survival gets primary attention. Only especially intact persons (and some senior professionals) are involved in, say, the national office of an agency serving the blind, the entertainment media, government, commercial sports (or the Olympics), the European Common Market, Interpol, a World Mental Health Congress, or the Board of IBM.

Perhaps you are wondering why the cosmic environment (Circle VI) is included. Every human being is affected by (the consequences of) the pull of gravity, sunspots, or great ideas (in the Platonic sense). The moon's impact on the tides, or the behavior of lovers, is well known. Today, the possibility that the full moon causes a rise in the incidence of hot-line telephone calls for help was studied by Lieber (1978). Also, a number of therapeutic approaches, such as those using meditation or yoga, emphasize the importance of being in harmony with the energies of the universe (Turner 1979).

According to this analysis, each of the environments in the model can contribute to (or hinder) a person's development and, in turn, can be influenced by this growing person. In order to help a client in distress, you may well have to intervene at many levels—as will be clarified.

The Family As Environment

In accordance with the model, the family is a person's first, and no doubt most significant, environment. Children raised by wolves can function as animals, but remain imperfect human beings. In fact, Portmann (1965) contends that human children emerge from the mother's physiological womb too soon (especially when compared to the newborn of other mammals).

He goes on to underscore the significance of the next nine months in "the social womb" of the family. In this womb, babies learn to sit, stand erect, trust, talk, walk, and even learn the rudiments of abstract thinking. This second set of nine months is so important that the human baby has to be expelled from the biological womb long before it is physically self-reliant.

The Participatory Environment

All individuals and families engage in relationships with nonkin persons, neighbors, peer groups, formal organizations, and intergroup collectivities such as public schools, churches, police, local stores, places of work, trade unions, well-baby clinics, day care centers, and Boy/Girl Scouts. Such services or agencies, each a complex organizational system, are located within the geographic neighborhood or within one's life space (Hall 1966, Watson 1970, Riemer 1959).

In the same way young men become tough Marines by participating in boot camp (Eisenhart 1977), all people are, in meaningful ways, products of the environmental units within which they are personally active during critical periods in their lives.

The Community Environment

Individuals, families, and complex organizations themselves become components of a larger collectivity—the community. In fact, Moe (1960) defined the community as a "system of systems." In the days of the Greek city-state, boundaries were geographically specific. However, whether small town or metropolis, the urban community is characterized by vague boundaries and seems more vulnerable to the impact of national level systems every year.

The "Distant" Environments

Systems analysis can be done for the three remaining environments in the model: the national, international, and cosmic. Although these impinge in important ways on the individual and the family, only relatively sophisticated people are aware of them. For most people, the family and the participatory environments are the world, and anything beyond them does not seem very important in daily life.

At the national level, you could analyze the functioning of such structural units as federations of labor unions, chambers of com-

merce, departments of government, head offices of voluntary agencies, etc. Internationally, you might benefit from a detailed systemic
study of the European Common Market, the United Nations, the
International Football Federation, OPEC, Interpol, etc., but these
efforts are beyond the purpose of this book.

Ecology: The System of Environments

Scholars of ecology use a very inclusive model of complex reality—open to physical and material things, people, social institutions,
information, and traditional values as well as new ideas (Emery and
Trist 1965). These scholars strive to coordinate a diversity of activities
scattered over a wide region and a high density of interacting units into
one macrosystem. As our technological capacity continues to develop
from human muscle power to animal power, wind and water power,
steam power, electric power, computer-television-telephone interfac-
ing, and nuclear power, the ecological scope of systems analysis is
becoming more and more important (Hawley 1979).

Today, practitioners at the level of regional ecosystems deal with
such broad issues as the humanization of metropolitan regions,
birth- and death-rate changes of large population groups, human
and animal migrations, preservation of the planet's ozone layer and
the purity of the oceans, and reversal of desertification in Africa
(Bennett 1976, Ophuls 1977). They rely on all the concepts of
systems analysis that are covered in the next chapters of this book.
In addition, they stress the capacity of open systems to adapt to
environmental changes or even innovate solutions to problems with
which other, less open systems are content merely to cope.

Ecologists are wary of tampering with only one item in any large
system. They know, for example, that the spraying of DDT against
mosquitoes or the use of pesticides by farmers can end up poisoning
entire food chains or underground water networks. All sorts of environmental problems are created when whole forests are cut down or
grasslands deteriorate: plants begin to die out, erosion occurs, and even
large watersheds dry up. Because there is little to eat, animals, birds,
and insects go elsewhere. When the local soil is no longer replenished
by their nutrients, the outcome is drought, uninhabitable deserts, large-
scale starvation, and even enforced mass migration (Ehrlich 1987).

Like other ecologists, Erlich advocates systemwide action that deals with all aspects of a deteriorating region simultaneously.

Germain (1973), in searching for new ways to redefine casework, utilized some ecological perspectives in the systems model she adopted. Specifically, she emphasized the interface between a person and the environment/milieu. She expects social caseworkers to promote growth-inducing experiences in the client's environment (e.g., a prenursery enrichment program) as well as offer direct counseling (to members of impoverished families). Many client difficulties are seen as arising from the inadequacy of housing, education, medical care, or from maldistributions of power in the environment.

As an ecologically oriented caseworker, Germain includes new service-delivery arrangements, volunteer and paraprofessional resources, and interdisciplinary consultations as part of the treatment plan. In 1978, Germain emphasized that the healthy ego takes an active and even creative role in adjusting to environmental changes such as physical migration or value shifts. Environmental nutrients and stimuli are seen as essential for the proper development of the ego throughout all stages of the life cycle.

In 1987, Germain further suggested that social workers abandon the still popular age-related models of human development and life transitions. She cites cohort theory, data on age and sex crossovers in postindustrial society, attachment theory, findings from research on normal infants, and longitudinal studies of handicapped children to make a strong case for growth models that do not rely on inflexible developmental sequences. Among her many sources, she cited Bronfenbrenner (1979), whose model focuses on the level of environmental complexity (from dyads to class and ethnicity groups) within which the growing individual interacts. She speculates about whether or not life transitions are essentially ecological ones.

EXPRESSING SYSTEM PRINCIPLES VISUALLY

In order to see how systemic variables interact (each influences the others and is influenced by them simultaneously), please study Figures 1.2 and 1.3. When two variables interact (e.g., husband and wife in a family system), the situation can be seen as two boxes joined by an arrow in both directions, or as two overlapping circles. As is pictured in Figure 1.2, these versions show that there are two relationships, and that there is a defined sub-area of common interests. Notice what happens when three variables (say a coalition of political parties) interact. In Figure 1.3, we can spot immediately that now there are six relationships. It is equally informative to see how there are three arenas in which only two of the variables interact, and one opportunity for the three of them to operate cooperatively.

As the number of factors or variables increases, so does the complexity of our system. Tools such as those above help us both to understand such complexity and to design effective ways of intervention in such a reality.

FIGURE 1.2. A Two-Item System

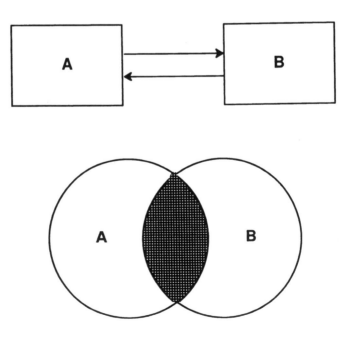

FIGURE 1.3. A Three-Unit System

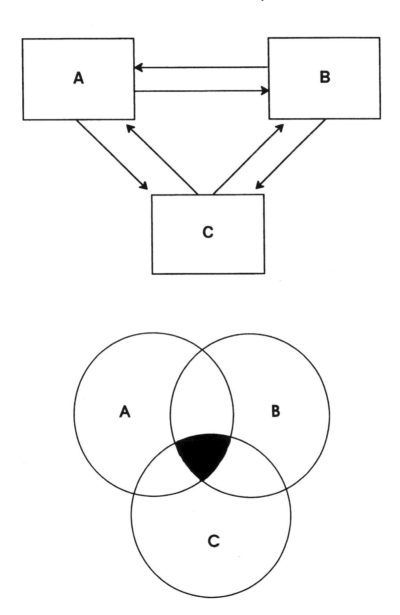

SUMMARY

You have been introduced to the idea of systems and to the possibility that systems analysis might be helpful in your social work practice. You were shown how to conceptualize a person as a social system and became acquainted with the six environments which surround every person. A section on ecology rounded out the chapter and helped you see how the client and the environment should be linked together in today's practice of social work.

It follows that any social unit can be analyzed as a system, as a component of a system, or as an environment (see Table 1.1). As you move from components to environments, your unit of analysis becomes more complex. In all instances, components, the system itself, and the environment regularly interact with one another. Specific exercises have been included to help you apply a systems approach to familiar situations.

Throughout this book, such multilevel analysis is used often. However, in order to be able to do this yourself, you will have to learn some of the basic concepts and characteristics of systems analysis. The next two chapters are meant to help you accomplish this goal.

TABLE 1.1. Components, Systems, and Environments as Units of Analysis

Components	Systems	Environments
Personality	Human being	Family or city
Human being	Family or peer group	M.H. Clinic or neighborhood
Family or neighborhood	Community or town	Ecological region or nation
Town or city	Nation or metropolitan area	NATO, EEC, or planet Earth

EXERCISES

Exercise 1: Environment Hopping

Please study the following example of multienvironment involvements.

> The tough, oldest son of a suburban family (who speak of him as their "black sheep") is making a lot of money pushing hard drugs in the high schools. He is a member of a criminal gang in his participatory environment while some of his victims, as participants in a drug-rehabilitation program, are struggling to "rid themselves of the habit." In the community and national environments, his activities are known as "organized crime" and are the targets of considerable police effort. Internationally, the World Health Organization, Interpol, and customs officials are fighting the "crack" trade. Some rehabilitated drug users might even speculate whether this "black sheep" is part of evil forces in the cosmos, or if he was born under an unlucky conjunction of stars and planets.

Using this model, fill in Table 1.2 with an example of your own. Using this multiple-environment model, try to analyze some person in your current work situation (male or female, young or old, majority or minority culture member, etc.). You might, for example, make up the profile of one of the "normal" relatives of the young man in the above example.

TABLE 1.2. Doing Some Multienvironmental Analysis

Environmental Level	Example of the "Black Sheep"	Your Example
Family:	Youngest son	_____
Participatory:	Drug pusher, gang member	_____
Community:	Criminal underworld	_____
National:	Organized crime	_____
International:	Mafia	_____
Cosmic:	"Evil stars and planets" (astrology)	_____

Exercise 2: Studying the Impact of Environments

Imagine a young man in the United States during the 1960s. Having just finished high school, he is facing induction into the army and is likely to find himself in the midst of the war in Vietnam. Even as a young person, he is already a Red Cross volunteer (having specialized in first aid) and hopes to go on to study medicine at a nearby college. On the other hand, he is being pressured by conflicting demands from various environments. For example:

> In the family environment, his father is a patriot. His mother does not want to "lose" her only son. Friends (from Canada) invite him to join them. Community institutions support and oppose the war. His country has just sent him a draft notice. News media continue to criticize the destruction in Vietnam.

If you were counseling such young adults back in the 1960s, what might you do to help one of them cope with these conflicting environmental demands?

Chapter 2

Some Characteristics of Open Systems

INTRODUCTION

Historically, Werner Lutz (1956) was among the first to suggest a systems model of social work practice. What he described as the "interactionist" model derives directly from a systemic approach to professional functioning. This model can be practiced in all social work settings and calls for an intervener with a holistic outlook. He particularly emphasized the multiorganizational or intersystemic nature of the environments in which our clients live and through which they are helped.

In order to examine such a possibility, it is important to learn some of the basic concepts of systems analysis. You can start by studying the P. family case record. It is used to illustrate such systems ideas as open/closed boundaries and vertical/horizontal relationships. Then, with the help of a second case history, you will look at the idea of positive and negative feedback as well as intersystem linkages. Toward the end of this chapter, you can review all these ideas by means of a detailed checklist to which you are invited to add your own examples.

HELPING THE P. FAMILY: A CASE REPORT

Imagine that you are responsible for helping the multiproblem P. family. You find the following in the agency's file:

The P. family was referred to our (mental health) clinic by their family physician because the 13-year-old son (Mark) continued to wet his bed every night despite many therapeutic attempts to help him. His parents, both in their late thirties, had immigrated from Italy as children. They married early and had four children: Mark, his two sisters Judy (age 16) and Catherine (age 8), and baby Freddie (age 2).

During the first interview, the social worker discovered that in addition to Mark's bed-wetting, the mother was tense about the father's inadequate income as a construction worker, and that the frequency of his staying in bed with backaches seemed to be increasing over the past months. Fights between the couple had escalated from loud shouts to physical violence. The family has other problems as well. The older daughter is deaf, and 8-year-old Catherine is failing in most of her school work. The P. family's extensive interaction with relatives and neighbors actually discouraged them from seeking social service help.

Amidst all these troubles, the caseworker noted that the family also possessed some strengths. Both parents were intelligent. The mother seemed to care deeply for the children (she was sufficiently motivated to accept casework help). The father, though unable to show much physical affection at home, demonstrated concern for the welfare of all family members. The basic strength of this family could be observed in the loving care everyone showed for baby Freddie (who was developing normally).

Although the mother agreed to come to appointments at the clinic, she often missed them, complaining that she could not get away because of her workload at home. The social worker decided to do the treatment through home visits. Because the father initially refused to participate, the worker responded to the wife's concern by visiting during a period when the father had been sick in bed for several days. His male self-image was threatened by the idea of talking to a female therapist about his work and physical problems, but he did go back to work the day after the worker's first visit. Thereafter, he participated occasionally in joint and family sessions, especially after fighting with his wife.

Over a period of three years of outreach casework treatment, family members improved their capacity to communicate with each other. The social worker initiated contacts with an agency for the deaf and the local public welfare office. Together they provided a special therapist to help the deaf older daughter.

While the social worker was helping the mother become less over-protective, the deafness therapist helped Judy increase her capacity to be active outside the home. The worker also initiated a conference between the mother and the teacher of the younger daughter, during which Mrs. P. was made to understand that her own behavior would have to change if Catherine's classroom work was to improve. After Mrs. P. began to trust Catherine to do her schoolwork on her own, the child's grades began to improve.

As the worker's support enabled the mother to feel less anxious, her talents as the family "go-getter" came into play. She explored the community and found her husband a job as a mail carrier, which fit his physical capacities much better. His attendance improved noticeably at this job, and he started talking about his "new friends from work." The ferocity of the marital fighting lessened, so that the mother spent less time running off to her own mother's home. The father and son were gradually freed from spending so much time caring for the youngest boy, Freddie, in her absence, and the lessened pressures at home helped both of them function better. Slowly and with occasional relapses, Mark woke up in a dry bed.

As you will see, this case contains a number of basic system concepts. After these concepts have been defined and illustrated, you should be able to apply them in your work as well as to help others do so appropriately.

DEFINITIONS AND CONCEPTS

Boundaries

Any systems analysis of the real world begins with an arbitrary definition of a boundary which separates what is inside the system from what is outside. At this stage of your knowledge of systems, if you focus on the P. family as a system, the parents, children, and perhaps a pet cat will be inside. The father's workmates, the neighbors, the grandmother, the clinic social worker, the schoolteacher, the public welfare office, the agency for the deaf, the family physician, the police, the landlord, and even the local grocery store owner are outside (or "out" in the system's environment).

Creating boundaries is a way to define a system. You can analyze the P. family as a social system within the neighborhood (its immediate environment). On the other hand, if you focus on the neighborhood as your system, the P. family becomes a component and the town becomes the environment. Similarly, if the mental health clinic in the P. family's case history is a system, it is embedded in an environment of municipal health services. If you let your imagination work, the clinic can also be an environment—when its outreach department is defined as the system. How the boundary is designated depends on what the analyst or intervener decides is most useful (Hearn 1970).

Hartman (1978, 1984, 1985) makes very practical use of boundaries in the child welfare field. Drawing on her knowledge of ecology, welfare, and psychology, she creates an *ecomap* to help workers and adoptive families assess strengths and limitations. This ecomap becomes a model for studying the complexity of internal relations as well as connections to various environmental bodies. It enables everyone to see the family as a dynamic totality and to analyze its boundary dynamics (i.e., the ease with which resources can flow from the environment, cross the boundary, and penetrate into the system). Relevant intervention strategies can also be mapped. In fact, the P. family situation might well be visualized with the help of such an ecomap (see Figure 2.1). You can check if you have grasped the idea of boundaries by trying Exercise 3, at the end of this chapter.

Thus, drawing the boundary is a way of analytically separating any system's internal components from its environment (Kirk 1972). Although interveners create boundaries for specific purposes, they are guided by knowledge and experience when doing so. Within an overall network of ongoing relationships, the boundary indicates a region of limited interaction (and, in a closed system, of no cross-boundary interaction). Boundaries can be relatively clear, as between an island and the surrounding ocean or between the P. family and the public school. Other boundaries are much more difficult to determine.

FIGURE 2.1. The P. Family Ecomap

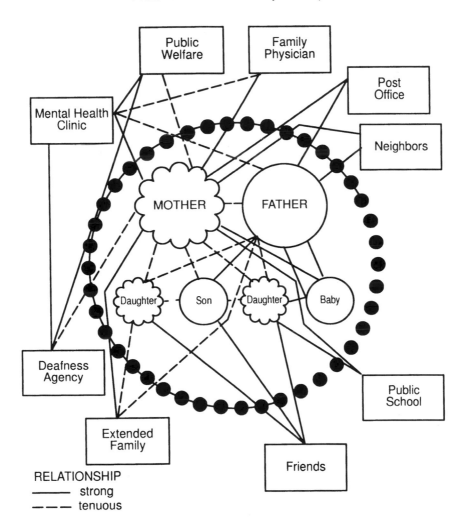

Perhaps the defining of a boundary is not altogether arbitrary. Table 2.1 gives you some clues. Units/actors within a cohesive system have a sense of so much in common that they strongly identify with each other. Relationships are personal, often intimate. These people are ready to share norms as well as power/resources and, with their sense of strong interdependence, will come to one another's aid

TABLE 2.1. Checklist for Clarifying System Boundaries

Individual's identification with the system is:	
1) Weak or absent ❏	2) Strong ❏
Interpersonal relationships are:	
1) Weak or absent ❏	2) Strong ❏
Sense of shared norms or values is:	
1) Weak or absent ❏	2) Strong ❏
Readiness to help one another is:	
1) Weak or absent ❏	2) Strong ❏
Power arrangements are:	
1) Assymetric ❏	2) Symmetric ❏
The boundary itself is seen as:	
1) Marginal ❏	2) Essential ❏

quickly. In fact, members of a multigenerational family (or residents of an ethnically homogeneous small town) often feel that a clearcut boundary not only strengthens their sense of identity and safety, but is vital for their survival. Boundaries do separate people "like us" from strangers (who are looked upon as untrustworthy). The walled towns of preindustrial Europe certainly gave their residents a feeling of belonging and security.

In contrast, environmental actors such as the police, welfare workers, teachers, store owners, and clerks at the agency for the deaf (outside the system's boundary), have less in common. When they do relate to each other, they usually do so on a pragmatic basis for the duration of dealing with a specific case or a collectivity. In the P. family example, the doctor, the mental health clinic, the public school, the public welfare agency, and the agency for the deaf each provide their specialized service—cooperating only when they happen to be serving the same client. These ideas are further clarified in the following section on open and closed systems.

Open and Closed Systems

A system is considered open if its boundary is relatively permeable; that is, when energy, information, or resources are exchanged with other systems in its environment (Allport 1960, Webber 1969). The rigid or relatively uncrossable boundary indicates a closed system, or one which tries to be totally independent from its environment.

For example, most religious cults try to build a closed boundary between themselves and their secular neighbors. In contrast, families in an ethnic neighborhood, where "everyone is like us," feel free to function in an open manner. Unlike the closed boundaries between Albania and its neighbors in the 1980s, relationships between Canada and the United States are characterized by open boundaries. Public schools, which are required to serve all children in their geographic area, have open boundaries. A private school, if it can be selective about whom it admits and is adequately financed from fees and private donors, may try to function like a closed system. Similarly, a catatonic schizophrenic, a slum area youth gang, or a bureaucratic department tend to behave in a closed manner.

Most systems involving human beings cannot be totally closed. In fact, since most human systems are made up of interacting smaller units, and since they also interact with other large units in their environment, tightly closed boundaries are unlikely. A humorous example of an open system is a domestic household in which the wife does the cooking and the husband takes out the garbage. The husband may be heard complaining—on the evening of the same day that he emptied all the garbage baskets, they are all filling up again. It might help to explain to him that the flow of garbage (an output) is one sign that the family's system is really open and is functioning effectively.

Professional practice, which holds that the world is composed of many open systems, would look at a problem holistically. In contrast, the reductionist approach seems to be based on a closed systems viewpoint. Thus, a counselor using a reductionist paradigm of the world would separate the P. family's troubles into manageable closed packages: those of the parents, the bed-wetting son, the deaf daughter, etc. Such an approach, clearly the opposite of the systemic one advocated in this book, has long been typical of services to multiproblem families. Our professional journals still complain that such families are treated in a fragmented (i.e., reductionist) way.

Two strategies can be used to counter such fragmentation. First, agencies responsible for dealing with one member or one specific aspect of a multiproblem family can learn to cooperate with other agencies serving the same family (see "systemic linkage" below). Second, the P. family, a partially closed system, can be helped to open up to various kinds of assistance from external agents. Based on an accurate diagnosis of the family's situation, strengthening the family included providing (inputs of) emotional support while opening its boundary so that it might receive help from various social services (Chin 1961, Goldberg and Neil 1972). This style of social work helped Mrs. P to improve her self-image, the son to stop wetting his bed, the deaf daughter to become more independent, the husband to suffer fewer backaches, and the younger daughter to improve her school grades, and lessened the quarreling between Mr. and Mrs. P.

Dependent or weak (partially open) systems are usually vulnerable to external influences. The P. family, like any weak or frail system, is likely to be exposed to pressures from social agencies, loan sharks, the police, etc., in its environment. In contrast, a very wealthy family can function with considerable independence of environmental pressures (i.e., in a relatively closed manner).

Boundaries may be objective, like those caused by geography, political loyalties, legal definitions, ethnic identity, etc. However, they can also be created artificially by labeling some person or group as inferior, or by imposing restrictions on their rights as was done to blacks and people of color in South Africa (Kuhn and Beam 1982). Such nonobjective boundary drawing, in which too-open or frail systems are exploited by powerful groups in their environment, underlies many of the problems that social workers are expected to deal with in their professional practice.

Vertical and Horizontal Interactions

Warren, Sanders, and many other writers on systems define certain interactions that take place within the system (i.e., between its components) as horizontal. Those that cross a boundary, or take place between two clearly defined systems, are considered vertical.

For example, members of a basketball team engage in horizontal relationships during practice. If they come before the discipline committee of the league because of some gross misconduct at a game, these relationships will be vertical.

If we hark back to Figure 1.1 in the first chapter (about individuals and environments), we can make some generalizations. Within each environmental circle (say, number III, the Community Environment), all the components of that circle/environment (e.g., City Hall, agencies, Chamber of Commerce, etc.) relate horizontally to each other. This is equally true of the relationships between the siblings within any one family (Circle I). When the Chamber of Commerce is engaged with the Manufacturers Association or with specific places of employment (in Circle II and IV), these relationships are considered vertical. The latter is also true of relations between a local school and the Ministry of Education (at the national level) or a store manager (his place of work) and the stock exchange (where he speculates).

In the P. family system, the relationships between the parents and their children and among the children would be called horizontal. Contacts between family members and the family doctor, the welfare department, the public school, or the agency serving deaf children would all be defined as vertical. In fact, the professional relationship used by the clinic's social worker to help the P. family over a period of years is essentially vertical. This worker also encouraged the family to develop new vertical contacts, in its environment, when such relationships were weak or did not exist.

Feedback

Healthy open systems must devote part of their resources to monitoring the impact of their outputs on their environment. Information thus obtained is used to make appropriate modifications in their ongoing internal behaviors. For example, classroom teachers (each of whom is a system) can check whether their outputs (lessons) are in fact enabling students (other systems in their environment) to learn. This is done by means of both informal feedback (students seeming interested or smiling) as well as formal feedback mechanisms (examinations). A similar process takes place between actors and audiences, officials and voters, etc. Figure 2.2 makes this process

FIGURE 2.2. Patterns of System-Environment Interaction

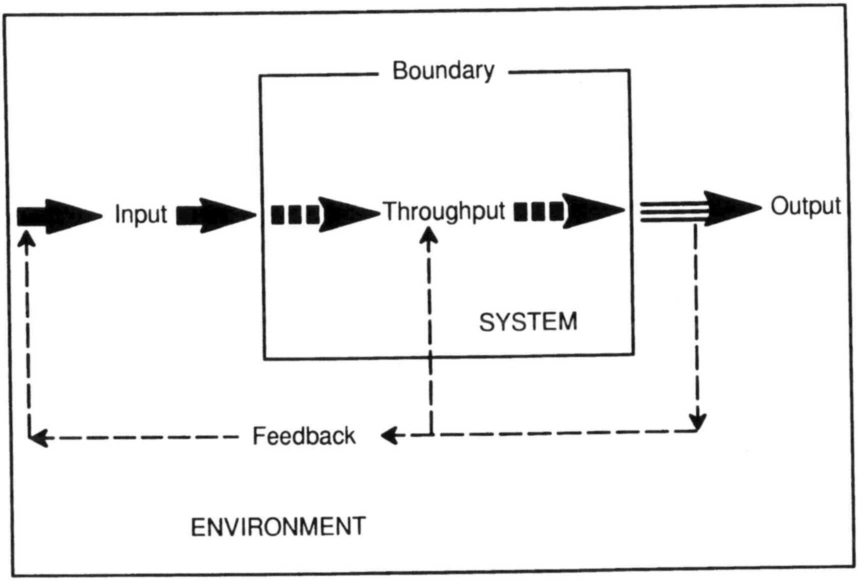

clear. Formal and informal response stimuli from the system's environment return through its boundary as feedback or as new inputs of information. Based on these messages, the system can adjust its efforts in order to achieve its goals more effectively (Kuhn and Beam 1982, Rosenberg and Brody 1974).

Feedback which confirms that the outcomes achieved are in line with our original intentions is called positive. We would probably continue what we have been doing or make an effort to increase our current inputs. On the other hand, feedback which indicates that our outcomes are unrelated to our original goals is called negative. This would caution us to reexamine what we have been doing and to look for alternative input efforts.

You can also utilize existing feedback patterns to explain some of the interaction between members of the P. family. When the classroom teacher first met with Mrs. P., the mother received some negative feedback, indicating that some P. family behaviors had to improve. As the son's bed-wetting decreased and the daughter's school grades improved (forms of positive feedback for their mother), Mrs. P's self-confidence increased. Support and approval (i.e., positive feedback) from the social worker enabled family members to stick with their new behaviors. Similarly, relative domestic peace, more trust from her mother, and special help from an agency in the environment (again, positive feedback), gave the deaf daughter enough self-confidence to venture out into the world on her own.

Social workers depend on the sensitive use of feedback for successful diagnosis as well as intervention. This includes skillful grasping of both the positive and negative feedback communicated by such actions as a smile, attentive or bored body posture, coldness or informality, silence or laughter, muscle tension or relaxation, etc. Such feedback sensitivity includes awareness that personal resistance or flaws in the environment can block feedback (i.e., communication) or distort it. If, after a few sessions of group therapy, client participation is enthusiastic (positive feedback), the social worker coleaders are likely to continue what they have been doing. If members of such a group, or of a group of young executives in an O.D. (organization development) training seminar, express boredom or stop attending (negative feedback), a change in format is called for.

Linkage

Creating links/connections between interacting systems or between components of one very large system is another idea basic to system-oriented practice. Such links are usually effective when exchanges among the different units or systems are two-way rather than when one system dominates the others. This is as true of marriage (the linkage of two one-person systems) as it is of a partnership (the linkage between two business organizations). Loomis (1959) described how rural and urban communities could function in a linked way for their mutual benefits. Linking systems and, perhaps, unlinking two systems when this becomes necessary (as in a divorce or in the dissolution of a business partnership) constitute important strategies of social intervention—as will be discussed later.

Lauffer (1982) suggests a number of processes used to create links among social agencies or professional helpers. As examples, he cites interagency case conferences, staff groups' adoption of joint standards or guidelines, sharing of expensive equipment, and standardization of reporting procedures for an entire field. Within a single agency, linking mechanisms include case management, staff meetings and consultations, and loaned staff arrangements. In the case history cited above, part of the clinic's success with the P. family is a result of the worker's skill in linking family members with relevant agencies, and in creating a modicum of cooperation among the various helpers.

In today's literature, making effective linkage is usually called networking. Accordingly, a staff person or a lay activist puts several persons and/or groups, who have been working independently toward a similar goal, in touch with each other and encourages them to proceed cooperatively in the future. Today, such results can be accomplished by means of computer links and electronic conferences that utilize two-way telephone-television technology. Another way to create linkage is to make certain that the same person (perhaps a supervisor) participates in a number of systems (e.g., by attending meetings of various staff groups, of supervisors, of the board, and of interagency representatives).

You might recall the many important linkage roles filled by Mrs. P. within her family system and by the clinic's social worker within the family's environment. Both women were able to serve linkage goals within the system, within the environment, and between the system and the environment. Creating such links may well be a therapeutically sound way to open up a family system that shows tendencies to function in a closed (i.e., defensive) manner.

SUMMARY

In order to review the concepts used in this chapter, look at the checklist in Table 2.2. Note that two columns have been filled with examples. The third column is left for you to complete regarding a system of your choice.

This systems-based model gives you tools for taking an orderly look at a total situation rather than dealing with small fragments. If you include such concepts as open systems or balanced combinations of vertical and horizontal relationships in your work, you will have taken the first steps toward a systems practice of social work. This includes improving your sensitivity to feedback and your skills

TABLE 2.2. First Review of System Concepts

Concept	Family Example	Welfare Office Example	Your Example
Systems boundary:	Kinship ties	Being an employee	_____
Open or closed:	Partially open	Partially open	_____
System components:	Parents and children	Staff and clients	_____
Units in the environment:	Welfare office clinic	National legislature	_____
		National office	_____
Horizontal relationships:	Parental fights	Staff meetings	_____
	Child-rearing	Coffee break	_____
Vertical relationships:	Counselor	National Association of Social Workers	_____
	Husband's employer		_____
Feedback via:	Bed wetting	Staff informality	_____
	Violence	Complaints	_____
Linkage via:	Love	Networking	_____
	Sharing	Exchanging	_____

in creating links. In addition, you will be able to sharpen your understanding of how subunits interact within a large unit (the system), and within a still larger unit (the environment). Any specific unit can be a component, a system, or an environment—especially when all the boundaries are open. As in Ezekiel's biblical vision, there are wheels within wheels "a-rollin'" dynamically and interacting in diverse ways.

In the coming chapters, you will learn additional concepts relevant to this systems-based model of practice. This systems model should also help you integrate knowledge from other practice models.

EXERCISES

Exercise 1: Drawing Boundaries

Draw a picture, similar to Figure 2.2, of the levels within your own work setting (for example, a family agency) as a system. Indicate the system's components, and show the other systems in your agency's environment with whom you interact regularly. The following two questions should help you get organized. Indicate what is inside your agency (the system), and what is outside its boundary.

Exercise 2: Identifying Open/Closed Systems

Using Table 2.3, give three examples each of open and of closed systems.

TABLE 2.3. Identifying Open and Closed Systems

Closed System	Example of Boundary
1) _____	_____
2) _____	_____
3) _____	_____
4) e.g., an island	e.g., the shoreline

Open System	Example of Boundary
1) _____	_____
2) _____	_____
3) _____	_____
4) e.g., the "P." family	e.g., kinship

Exercise 3: Identifying Horizontal/Vertical Interactions

Using Hartman's type of ecomapping (explained above), and basing yourself on the P. family story, give some examples of relationships that would be defined: (a) as horizontal; and (b) as vertical. Based on your own professional experience, repeat this exercise, giving examples of vertical and horizontal relationships in a treatment group or in a voluntary association.

Exercise 4: Analyzing a Feedback Problem

Liberal members of the Parent-Teachers Organization of a school located in an upper middle-class (white) suburb decided that they wanted their grade eight pupils to make contact with black children of the same age. If it could be an educationally sound experience, such meetings should help prepare both groups to appreciate each other and to work together for peaceful coexistence during their adult years.

They understood that this sort of project required the cooperation of a black school's principal and teachers, some parents, and perhaps an influential person such as a church leader. The nearest black neighborhood with an appropriate counterpart school proved to be just over the city line, on the outskirts of the metropolitan region. After a round of consultations, the suburban school wrote a letter to the principal of the counterpart school requesting a meeting with him in order to explore the feasibility of a joint activity.

Three days later, before they had received an answering letter, one of the teachers of the suburban school was surprised to receive a phone call from a teacher-colleague of the city school. She had met him at a recent workshop and both had admired each other's teaching skills. The caller (a black male) seemed enthusiastic about the prospect of planning a joint educational day. In contrast, the suburban teacher (a white woman) became uncomfortable with her colleague's unexpected invitation to come to his home for a cup of coffee that evening and chat informally about the project. Even though he promised to arrange for the attendance of his school's principal and PTO chairperson, the white teacher replied that she could not come to the session since she had to check with her PTO chairperson and her principal. She would call him back in a few days.

List some of the informal feedback examples that appear in the above story, adding your own opinion regarding what each feedback message contributed to the advance or the delay of the project. For example:

Feedback 1: The black teacher invited his white colleague to an informal evening meeting at his home. He seemed to be giving positive feedback to the message his school had received in the letter.

Its impact: Even though she was liberal about black-white cooperation, she felt uneasy about going to a black man's home by herself.

Feedback 2:_____

Its impact:_____

Feedback 3:_____

Its impact:_____

In light of the indication that the white teacher could not speak for her PTO or for her principal, what might be the content of the black principal's letter of reply (to be sent by the end of the week)?

When the white teacher telephoned back a few days later, what might she have told her black colleague in order to enhance the prospect of black cooperation in this project?

Chapter 3

Additional Characteristics of Open Systems

INTRODUCTION

In the previous chapter, you learned some of the basic concepts of systems analysis. This chapter continues the process. A multi-environment case history, that of Betty D., will provide a concrete example for the new concepts to be learned. A summarizing checklist will give you another opportunity to review and to fill in a blank column regarding an example of your choice.

THE BETTY D. SITUATION: A CASE REPORT

Betty D., a 52-year-old married mother of three children, has an MBA from a prestigious college and a good job. For reasons she finds difficult to explain, she has felt increasingly irritable during the past few months, and arthritic pains have begun bothering her. Understandably, she spends many hours each week searching for ways to get relief from her pain.

Betty is aware of tension in three major areas of her life:

1. *At work* (her participatory environment). As one of two comptrollers in a local textile plant, her tension/anger was alienating many colleagues. Lately, her employer asked her to retire early—ostensibly because the plant has been losing sales and must cut back economically.

2. *At home* (her family environment). Almost every day, she is caught up in shouting arguments with her husband (a

salesman who travels extensively) or her teenaged daughter, recently suspended from high school for taking drugs. She also finds herself in frequent conflict with her long-time neighbors (within her participatory environment).

3. *At City Hall* (her community environment). For the past eight years, Betty has served as consultant to the mayor on matters of finance and administration, but the quality of her advice has become inconsistent during the past year. Also, her ability to persuade members of City Council is on the decline.

Using reductionist models, you might approach this situation by separating Betty's troubles into manageable packages: intrapersonal (psychiatric), interpersonal (social work relationships), organizational (labor-management relations), communal (sociology/political science), etc. Treatment based on one or another of these approaches would be fragmented according to profession or type of agency specialization. In contrast, if relying on a systems model, you would look at the D. family as an open system that suffers from internal malfunctions and conflicts with other systems in its environment. Ideally, an intervener would analyze Betty's situation in its entire personal-organizational-community complexity (see Figure 3.1).

If you concentrate an the D. family system, Betty's neighbors, workplace, City Hall, etc., are parts of the environment. Her husband, daughter, various biological-psychological conditions, and Betty herself are components of the family system. She experiences negative reactions from the horizontal relationships with her husband and daughter as well as from her vertical involvements at work, in the neighborhood, and at City Hall. The daily accumulation of negativity in her life may well be feeding her tension and worsening her arthritis.

Using systems concepts enables you to intervene by drawing different sets of boundaries. Suppose you decide to focus on Betty's work setting as the system. If so, her supervisor, various colleagues, and other departments at the plant become system components (horizontal relations), and family troubles are out in the environment (vertical relations). Her superiors might well reason that Betty's difficulties with her neighbors, arthritic pains, and domestic troubles

FIGURE 3.1. Betty D.'s Multiple Environments

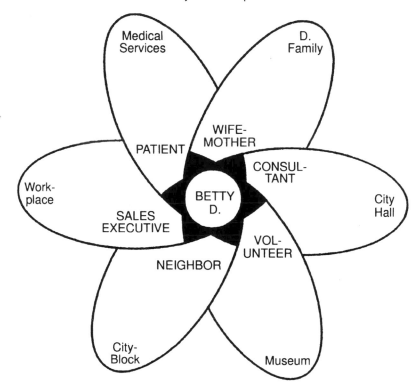

are interfering with her work. With Betty's consent, a systems-oriented worker would probably try to coordinate the efforts of a team of psychological, medical, and organizational development (O.D.) helpers simultaneously in order to help Betty effectively (Chin 1961, Goldberg and Neil 1972).

As in the previous chapter, this case study will serve as a vehicle for learning a few more basic concepts from systems analysis.

MORE DEFINITIONS AND CONCEPTS

Input, Throughput, Output

In order to maintain themselves, systems seek (and constantly absorb) resources such as food, stimulation, energy, raw materials, love, money, advice, information, ideas, equipment, fuel, etc., from the outside through a permeable border. For example, when Betty studied at business college, various environments provided her with such *inputs* as food, lectures, library, housing, grades, etc. Similarly, an agency or clinic (organizational) system seeks such inputs as clients, budget, personnel, and enabling policies in order to survive. Whatever form they take, inputs or resources must be sufficient— and of high enough quality—not only to sustain the system but also to provide it with enough of an energy surplus for growth and some experimentation.

Coherent systems (defined at the end of this chapter) use their inputs by employing such *throughput* processes as digesting food, thinking about ideas, coping with stimuli, managing within available budget, and the like. As a result, the system generates *outputs* (e.g., services, reports, products, "alumni") which are exported across its boundary into the environment to become the inputs of another system. For example, Betty's daughter, the output of a family system, becomes the input of a public school (organizational) system. Similarly, Betty's output of expert advice becomes an input in the mayor's decision making at City Hall.

In every situation or environment, the outputs of one system become the inputs of another, making it possible for systems to exchange goods, information, or relationships for their mutual benefit (Heath 1976). Humans and other animals breathe out carbon dioxide, an unwanted output, which is used by plants, an essential input for photosynthesis. The plants, in turn, produce oxygen (their unneeded output) which is an essential input for human metabolism. The textiles produced by Betty's factory become merchandise sold by a local store to customers who buy cloth to make curtains for their bedrooms, etc.

Similarly, the funds raised by a United Way campaign become, after a careful allocation process (throughput), the inputs of agencies such as Family Service or the YMCA. The annual service reports of these agencies become public relations materials that the United Way uses to campaign for additional funds next year. And the cycle continues—hopefully in a positive, steady state.

You may also encounter the phenomenon of "input overload." This refers to a system that is so overwhelmed with inputs that it becomes paralyzed. In times of community emergency, such as an earthquake, even telephone hot lines can become so overloaded with cries for help that they cease to function altogether (Drabeck and Haas 1969). Small agencies, for instance, a person who wins a high-purse sweepstake, can prove incapable of deciding how to spend a large new income. Instead, they just limp along as they did in former days of minimal resources, with which they are familiar.

Betty D.'s outputs are as negative as her inputs. She is now known for her outbursts of anger and the inconsistent quality of her professional advice, causing others to avoid her and even to complain about her performance. She is losing her influence at City Hall—all this while feeling overloaded. As she copes less and less adequately, her tension is likely to increase.

Equilibrium, Homeostasis, Growth

Because these three concepts refer to the differing degrees of a boundary's openness, Anderson and Carter (1974) found it useful to make clear distinctions between them.

Equilibrium

A closed system, having a fixed structure and no vertical interaction with its environment, experiences horizontal relationships only. Such a system creates its own (internal) equilibrium. For example, a chemical reaction within a clearly enclosed space will eventually reach a state of equilibrium and be seen as stable. If some external force (e.g., heat) manages to penetrate the boundary, the system absorbs this impact, either returning to its former equilibrium or establishing a new one. Thus, hydrogen and oxygen, sparked with electricity within a closed space, combine to create a specific quantity of water. If enough heat is added from the outside, the new equilibrium will be at the boiling point of water, but the water remains unchanged.

Many bureaucratic organizations or elitist social groups act as if they are in a state of equilibrium (i.e., closed to their environment). Families with a deformed child sometimes try to hide behind closed boundaries. Similarly, members of a stigmatized minority group in a hostile majority culture (or a severely paranoid individual) often defend themselves against inputs from other systems in their environment by functioning in an equilibrium manner.

Homeostasis

On the other hand, homeostasis, or steady state, refers to open systems. Homeostasis is used to describe a system that is in constant interchange with its environment (e.g., a lake which maintains a constant level by receiving water from melting snows and releasing excess waters over a spillway). The result may seem stable, but is a dynamic balance and not a static equilibrium. Most normal relations include give and take or homeostasis with colleagues at work, neighbors, and loved ones. In her good days, Betty D. must have functioned in this manner.

Growth

Finally, the term growth is used to describe an open system which not only exchanges with its environment but is capable of altering its structure in order to adapt to changing conditions (Lewin 1961). In this situation, the system's throughputs also undergo a change. Healthy persons, organizations, groups, and even cultures are seen as seeking challenges (Maslow 1954, Jantsch 1981). Open systems create new functions or internal structures as a part of their potential for self-transformation, self-healing, self-renewal, or internally stimulated evolution. A growth capacity is considered basic to all living systems. Healthy open systems do not aim for stability or concentrate only on need reduction. Rather, they see tension, strain, or conflict as wholesome because these create the necessity for coping and function as a precondition for growth (i.e., for raising the system to a higher level of maturity).

Thus, older adults who face retirement within a continuing person-environment interchange are likely to survive this transition. They learn new hobbies, develop new friendships, and undertake new roles—all above and beyond having to make healthy adjustments to specific losses during their remaining years. In contrast, Betty D.'s condition is deteriorating. She is unable to defend herself by withdrawing (i.e., by becoming a more closed system). In fact, her person-environment situation is beyond maintaining itself as either a closed equilibrium or a homeostatic give-and-take.

COMMUNICATIONS
AND SYSTEM-ENVIRONMENT RELATIONS

At this point, a systems-based model of normal communications between two parties might help you understand the dynamics of boundary crossing (Nowotny 1981). Please examine Figure 3.2 carefully. Entering a two-unit communication network arbitrarily at phase 1, information source A initiates some recognized behavior (e.g., sits down to write a report). He/she arranges letters of the alphabet into a pattern of words and syntax (or encodes meaning into this *throughput* activity), and creates a message. When A makes a further effort to transmit it (e.g., goes to the post office and mails the report to B), the message becomes A's *output*. The letter is then injected into some

FIGURE 3.2. Cycle Flow of Interunit Communication

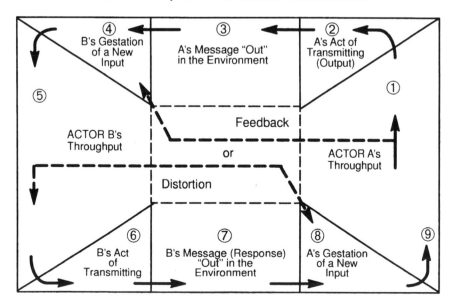

external medium or *environment* (e.g., the mails). If it is properly routed, and if nothing interferes or offers resistance, the transmission will probably arrive at its destination (although it may help to send the report by express or registered mail). In phase 4, when the message is received, it becomes B's *input*. It then undergoes decoding, and hopefully conveys both meaning and feeling to the receiver. If, as is usually the case, a response is indicated, B's reply goes through a similar set of steps (from 6 to 8) in order be transformed into A's *input*.

During the entire cycle, meaning can be lost if:

1. A's encoding or transmission is faulty (e.g., unclear handwriting or forgetting the zip code),
2. either the sender or the receiver lets emotions such as fear or anger interfere with their concentration,
3. the environment is clogged (e.g., by the Christmas overload of mail), or
4. B's system of decoding is different from the one used by A.

Should A and B meet on the street during this time, they might shorten the process by making a comment, asking a question, smiling or frowning—providing *feedback* (arrows from 3 to 8, 7 to 4). Of course, the feedback will not help if it is inaccurate, distorted, or misinterpreted.

This analysis can be applied to the interaction between a husband and wife, a neighborhood association and City Hall, or a county welfare service and the relevant state or national department or ministry. Such analysis becomes useful for explaining what happened between members of the P. family and the mental health clinic in its (participatory) environment (see Figure 3.3).

In an adaptation of the communications cycle model, A (from Figure 3.2) has become Mrs. P. (the mother-wife of a troubled family), and B is the mental health clinic. With the help of her physician, Mrs. P.'s problem was transmitted to the mental health clinic, and a worker was assigned to help her. As is common, her expression of need was translated by clinic staff into a request for specific services (or service changes) as it traveled through the channels that linked the client to the appropriate helping agency. Thus, in phase 4, agency personnel decoded her message in terms of

FIGURE 3.3. Application of the Communications Cycle

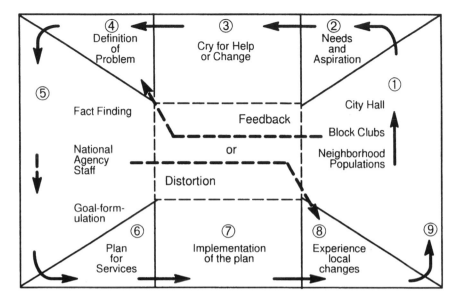

medical, counseling, linkage, or welfare problems. This did approximate the needs of Mrs. P. at that time.

The clinic's workers and supervisors most likely put the message through such additional subprocesses as fact finding, diagnosis, consultation, staff brainstorming sessions, etc., before formulating service goals for the case. In phase 6, policy goals were transformed into a plan for offering a package of services. The latter were implemented in various ways by many professional intervenors. In phase 8, members of the P. family personally experience or observe behavioral changes taking place, and this becomes new input for their continuing into a second cycle of communication. In the latter, they may communicate directly, or by means of feedback, an expression of satisfaction or protest—and the second cycle is rolling.

If you recall, Mrs. P. was not showing up for appointments at the clinic, thus blocking the flow of communication. The worker diagnosed Mrs. P. as suffering from a low self-image but with sufficient strengths to respond positively to therapy. She decided on an outreach approach which culminated in a series of therapeutic home visits, unblocking the communication between Mrs. P. and the clinic. Perhaps your analysis of the above communications model should include such familiar concepts as process, support, insight, diagnosis, outreach, home visits, and self-image.

FUNCTIONS

Many anthropologists and sociologists agree that, for efficient systems analysis, it is important to understand how different components of any system contribute to the survival of the total entity. A function refers to a process or activity essential to a system's continuity. In the P. family, the mother initially felt that strict control of her children (see "social control" below) was essential for their normal growth and development.

Kirk (1972) clarifies the usefulness of this kind of analysis by explaining that client behavior which seems deviant (e.g., heavy drinking) may actually contribute to the person's overall mental balance. Similarly, Navaho acceptance of witchcraft can be functional (or effective) for individuals as well as for the overall society in which they live. In traditional Navaho society, witchcraft can explain how to become wealthy, dispose of enemies, find an outlet for strong aggressiveness, sublimate antisocial tendencies, or gain attention (Kluckhohn 1944, Merton 1957).

When a behavior does not serve a vital purpose or seems detrimental to a system's survival, it is described as dysfunctional. Becoming addicted to hard drugs is dysfunctional for the users, their families, and other systems in their environment. Similarly, a violent tornado or race riots usually prove dysfunctional for a community.

While analyzing broad social changes in the United States in 1963, sociologist Roland Warren suggested that five functions are essential to every community system. These include production-distribution-consumption, socialization, social control, mutual support, and social participation. Warren's model can, in fact, be applied to all open systems. Thus, components of any system perform one or more of the five essential functions as elaborated below.

Production-Distribution-Consumption

This function guarantees that essential goods and services are produced and eventually reach systems that consume them (as inputs). If the father in the P. family works, his income becomes available for buying food and clothes for his wife and children (assuming that farms and factories have produced these items from raw materials, and that they have been distributed to local stores and supermarkets). Similarly, collected taxes pay for social security benefits or public parks. In fact, many conservative governments subsidize private industry rather than let bankruptcy initiate a vicious cycle of large-scale unemployment followed by less income available for consumption, less demand, less production, and so on into a recession.

In the welfare state, a family lacking a stable source of income must rely on public assistance, rent subsidies, subsidized medical care, food stamps, or other substitute money sources in order to continue existing in a consumer economy. Similarly, a day care center for the aged builds its budget from user fees, municipal payments for service, philanthropic gifts, sales of paintings done by participants, etc. In both cases, of course, if the cupboard is bare, the system falters.

Socialization

This refers to the means by which new recruits are found for the system and how these newcomers are taught the values and behavioral expectations essential to becoming an accepted member. For example, a traditional family socializes its children to stay within their ethnic culture by means of modeling, positive reinforcement, and selective use of sanctions. A professional school initiates a "lay" person into the role behaviors of a social worker through formal lessons, guided experiences, grades, and the like. Everyone in a given culture is "carefully taught" how to be a patient in a hospital, how to be a recipient of charity, and even how to accept the majority group's stereotypes.

These days, socialization is accomplished, to varying degrees, by such actors or systems as the family, clergy, television, self-help groups, traffic police, youth gangs, political parties, voluntary associations, partisans of various ideologies, and the public schools. When their messages reinforce each other, they tend to make for a stable community or society. If these agents of socialization clash, growing young persons or immigrants are likely to suffer serious difficulties.

Social Control

Social control helps keep a system's subunits in line after they have become legitimate members of the system. Control is usually achieved through rewarding desired behaviors and punishing those which are considered deviant. For example, in a rural village or small town, the gossip chain restrains deviance effectively while recognition from a church elder rewards the faithful. In metropolitan society, police, legislation, and government are instruments of social control. In most professions, ethics committees (negative sanctions) and publication opportunities (positive reinforcements) accomplish this outcome.

In native (American and Canadian) societies, a circle of elders works with local deviants in order to understand, and then to correct, disturbing behaviors (such a circle seldom resorts to shame or punishment, although insufferable deviants are sometimes excommunicated). In current urban society, ADR (alternative dispute resolution) techniques are becoming popular. Increasingly, judges are sending specific types of "criminals" to mediation rather than sentencing them to a period in jail.

Mutual Support

This function provides members of a social system with ways to help each other or assist someone who is not self-sustaining. Rural extended families and/or neighbors once helped each other in times of need through such mechanisms as the husking bee or barn raising. Religious charitable efforts helped to marry off the daughters of poor families, ransom captives, maintain indigent elders, give support during times of mourning, etc. In modern days, mutual support mechanisms include cooperatives, voluntary social agencies, public welfare and other government-sponsored social services, self-help groups/networks, philanthropic foundations, and the United Way. Both the helping professions and social service bureaucracies implement this function in the welfare state of today.

Social Participation

Participation refers to the ways people are able to become involved (horizontally) in the decision making of a human system as well as gain a strong sense of belonging to the system. Participation is made possible through such mechanisms as committees, boards or councils, communal church worship, protest movements, serving at the precinct level of a political party, or volunteering in social agency settings. The famed War on Poverty advocated maximum feasible participation by residents from impoverished neighborhoods in planning the programs that affected their daily lives.

Certainly, one way to bring about a change in a community service's policies is to include a substantial number of local residents on the board of directors, along with the usual people of power and influence. As elaborated in a coming chapter, opportunities to participate are crucial for resolving many types of conflict.

MANIFEST AND LATENT FUNCTIONS

You may have noticed that there is often a gap between officially recognized (manifest) functions and what really goes on (the latent function). Merton (1957) explains how a formal ceremony, whose historical origins have been lost over the years, may still serve the latent function of participation, thereby giving group members a continuing sense of belonging and safety. Even though the manifest function of a local public welfare office is mutual support, its unofficial function is often social control of the community's poor.

Most suburban grade schools function effectively in the field of socialization, and high percentages of their graduates finish high school or go on to study at a university. Some schools are known for their additional commitment to the participation function, accomplished by means of student councils, pedagogic councils, parent committees, and interdisciplinary conferences about problem children. Other schools, especially those in slum areas, function as social controllers. For them, keeping "problem" kids off the streets is preferable to the clashes of violent street gangs.

In light of the above, a systems-oriented therapist would try to clarify how Betty D.'s tension and arthritis are affecting her life. Along with relevant colleagues, at a case conference, they would use their diagnostic powers to identify the causes of her current discomforts. According to Warren's model of system functions, Betty seems to be endangering her ability to earn a salary (production), losing her influence at City Hall (participation), and setting a very negative example of socialization for her daughter. This also causes her to provide her daughter with lessened inputs of parental love and guidance. In order to help, the same therapist might activate a consultant from within Betty's work setting (the production-distribution-consumption function) to help her improve relations with colleagues and subordinates as well as cope with the threat (social control) of early retirement. Simultaneously, health and social work (mutual support) professionals would counsel her concerning her arthritis while helping her family. After her energy level improves, recruiting Betty into a small neighborhood project (participation) might prove useful. In general, all members of the D. family may have to undergo a basic resocialization before they are able to improve their behaviors within the family system and/or out in its environment.

Did you notice that, within an urban-industrial community or national system, one structure can accomplish a number of different functions, and a number of different structures can produce the same function? For example, in Exercise 9 (at the end of this chapter), Blue Cross carries out four functions while both it and the police provide mutual support. It is also useful to specify for whom the function is done. The police, for example, socialize when they teach traffic safety in grade schools. They execute social control when they arrest traffic violators, and they offer mutual support when they rush a poverty-stricken pregnant woman to the hospital. The same phenomenon is summarized for both rural and urban communities in Table 3.1.

TABLE 3.1. Systemic Functions in Two Types of Communities

Systemic Function	Examples of Functions in	
	Village	**Metropolis**
Economy	Barter at the market	Banks, stock market
	Hard Labor	Subsidies
	Many children guarantee needed manpower	Many children are a costly consumer liability
Socialization	The family	Public schools, television
	The church	Military service
	Apprenticeship	Professional school
Social Control	Neighborhood gossip	Police, courts, law
	Excommunication	News media expose
	Visit the county fair	Receive the keys to the city
Mutual Aid	Personal help to the needy	Bureaucratized welfare office
	Neighborhood barn raising	Federal disaster relief
	Poor law	Social security
Participation	Local politics	Neighborhood association
	Church clubs, fraternal groups	Neighborhood center's Board of Directors
	Town meeting discussions	Public opinion survey, referendum

COHERENCE

In addition to all the above characteristics, members of open systems are held together by a kind of internal (social-emotional) glue. They survive by having been socialized into a web of shared expectations-norms-values (e.g., to respect their elders), kinship or friendship ties, obligations to help each other in times of trouble, loyalties, mutual role expectations (e.g., how husbands and wives should behave), and the like. Common historical memories (e.g., surviving slavery, winning a war of independence) or shared current experiences (e.g., the excitement of a national sports event, suffering through a disaster together) also help the system's members achieve emotional coherence.

Open systems can be strengthened by improving the coherence mechanisms of the system. This is helped if the system has a steady surplus of inputs over outputs so that resources are available for both promotion of internal growth as well as high-risk experiments. Coherence is increased when members of a system (e.g., the Police Athletic League) receive positive feedback regarding the successful contribution their outputs (volunteering to run basketball leagues) are making to the welfare of other systems in the environment (the lessening of juvenile delinquency). Coherence may also be strengthened when the system's components (e.g., the eight members of an agency staff) share enough positive group experiences to develop a "we feeling." This is often the natural result of opportunities within the participation function.

Despite all their troubles, the D. family system remains intact because Betty and other family members share remembrances of an earlier, happier time, and because basic loving relationships still exist. Family, religious, and community rituals may also be helping the system to stay together. If these are absent, the family might well split apart in divorce, or Betty might be removed from it by a prolonged hospitalization.

REVIEW OF THE SYSTEMS MODEL

As part of getting acquainted with systems analysis, you have been learning many new concepts. At this point, you should also be able to apply these concepts to a range of micro- and macrosystems. The rest of this chapter allows you to consolidate these new learnings and to practice using them.

The Individual As a System

As noted earlier, the individual human being can be conceptualized as a system. A person is composed of many components or subsystems. The basic one is, of course, the biological body. Its skin is a boundary with the environment, and its many component organs and metabolic processes are crucial for the continuation of life. Second, the human individual has functions intellectually—

learns (through cognitive efforts, scholarship, structured experiences of socialization, etc.) and transfers such learnings to new situations. This component also makes empirical studies possible, with the assistance of our senses, and enables us to enjoy logical reasoning.

Third, no human person can function without feelings, emotions, or the nonintellectual capacity called intuition. We can do without jealousy or hatred, but love and fear and anger are basic to human behavior, and a range of emotions lies behind the beliefs and values to which we are committed. Fourthly, many contemporary scholars are convinced that any healthy or complete person also functions on a spiritual level.

The above four components alone make the human being into a complex system. Of course, outside this system's boundary lies an equally complex environment. It is made up of a physical ecology, social environments as well as the all-embracing system called tradition. These are all sources of inputs for the developing human being and constitute some of the settings in which personal outputs are absorbed by other systems.

The Family Environment/System

As you know from Figure 1.1, the family itself can be analyzed as an *open* system, exchanging in a steady way with diverse elements in its *environment*. A nuclear family usually includes the parents, small children, and, perhaps, a dog. *Horizontal relationships* flow along generational, male-female, or sibling lines while each family member also engages in a diversity of *vertical relationships* with other families, work colleagues, fellow students, church members, Boy/Girl Scouts, other dog lovers, medical clinic staff, informal friendship groups, etc., in the environment.

Parental salaries and other sources of family income are important *inputs*—as are the values, norms, and role expectations which stem from religious traditions, membership in social class and ethnic groups, reference groups, television, etc. Family *throughputs* include making decisions about spending or saving money, what style of clothing to wear, how to raise the children, where to live, where to go for summer vacation, what religious practices to observe, or how to care for aging grandparents. Just as the parents' marriage linked two family systems, the older son's romance is likely to create another *linkage* between his family and that of his fiancée. The children as well as the furniture produced by parental efforts, at home or in a factory, are *outputs* that are hopefully enriching or useful to other family systems in the vicinity.

Although the family still has primary responsibility for *socialization* of children, today it is assisted by the mass media, community centers, the public schools, churches, etc., in its environment. *Social control* is accomplished by means of positive and negative reinforcements as well as police and law courts. Family members engage in *mutual aid*, but (again) are helped by many educational, health, and welfare agencies. Internally or environmentally generated crises, which may upset a system's balance temporarily, are often *functional* forerunners of growth spurts. Report cards from school, promotions at work, and neighborhood recognition (for leadership) are forms of *feedback* that help the family system redirect the behavior of its members.

The Environment/System We Participate in Personally

Again following the environment model of Figure 1.1, family members normally become involved in such components of their participatory environment as service organizations, night clubs, workplaces, shopping centers, etc. As in the systems analysis of a family (above), local service organizations—if thriving on inputs such as money, manpower, equipment, or raw materials of sufficient quantity and reasonable quality—will ensure participation opportunities for neighborhood residents.

Each organization processes its own throughput so that the above inputs are converted into such outputs as lessons, interviews, vaccinations, advice, money allowances, protection, hospitalization, tennis courts, organized trips, specific jobs, repair services, etc., for various audiences of consumers or participants. As a way of keeping track of how well it is doing, each organization should also make use of feedback reports from its clients-consumers-participants, governmental regulatory bodies, staff, market research teams, and competitors.

The Community Environment/System

Subsystems or components of the community system include voluntary social agencies, clinics, a chamber of commerce, local chapters of various political parties, a public welfare office, public schools, banks, department stores, churches, and neighborhoods (Bebout and Bredmeier 1963, Sanders 1975). In this environment, for example, socialization is the partial or complete output of the family, neighbors, peer groups, reference groups, ethnic groups, public and private schools, workplaces, local television, churches, etc.

Most of the organizations in the community environment, like the individuals in a family environment, are caught up within a network of horizontal and vertical relationships, thereby experiencing many exchanges with other systems and environments. As an open system, a welfare office will likely be involved horizontally with grade schools, a health clinic, the police, employment agencies, the fire department, etc., in caring for the same multiproblem family. It is also tied vertically to its own regional and/or national offices as well as a legislature, for policy guidelines, and a treasury, for budget.

Most communities are held together by a number of systemwide coherence structures. These include the following:

1. A stable power structure and shared respect for all authorities
2. Sufficient economic inputs to guarantee a basic level of subsistence and public services for all persons and groups of the community
3. Shared historical experiences (past inputs)
4. Integrating/coordinating structures like a church federation, a chamber of commerce, a board of education, political coalitions, or a council of social agencies
5. A sense of common values, norms, and expectations that sometimes take the form of a tradition or ideology which makes things legitimate

6. Effective feedback processes (mirrored in voter turnout, complaints to the mayor or local ombudsman, letters to the editor, public opinion polls, etc.) that prevent dissatisfaction from escalating into rumors, hysteria, or rioting
7. A social "atmosphere" in which expressing emotions is acceptable and wins a measure of appropriate support

SUMMARY

In order to review the concepts used in this chapter, please look at Table 3.2. Again, two columns have been filled with examples. The third column is left for you to complete regarding a system of your choice.

TABLE 3.2. Second Review of System Concepts

Concept	Family Example	Welfare Office Example	Your Example
Growth:	Maturation	Agency expansion	_____
Equilibrium:	Fanatic	Bureaucracy	_____
Input:	Groceries	Budget	_____
Throughput:	Make meals	Hire staff	_____
Output:	Husband's work	Monthly checks	_____
Socialization:	Public school	Staff workshop	_____
Social control:	Parental praise	Supervision	_____
Mutual support:	Counseling	Coffee break	_____
Participation:	Shared tasks	Staff committee	_____
Coherence:	Cultural tradition	Professional values	_____

By now you know that any proper definition of a social system has to include the following:

1. Arbitrary, clearly designated boundaries
2. Within these boundaries, a set of persistent, functionally inter-dependent (horizontal) relationships among the components of the system
3. Beliefs, sentiments, symbols, and control mechanisms that reinforce the system's coherence and persistence
4. A contextual or external environment that includes a set of interacting (other) systems
5. Some system components that have various vertical relation-ships with components of other systems in the environment
6. Continuous interchange of relationships or resources among the components of a system, as well as between them and the system's environment

Once familiar with these concepts, you should be ready to examine the ways in which systems analysis can both help social workers understand social change and supply them with additional technology for bringing about planned change.

EXERCISES

Exercise 1: Identifying Inputs, Throughputs, and Outputs

In thinking about your family or an agency within which you have worked, list examples of the three processes described above using Table 3.3. In either case, are the inputs and the throughputs adequate so as to leave a surplus for growth? Whether your answer is yes or no, describe this situation in a paragraph or two.

TABLE 3.3. Input, Throughputs, and Outputs

Family Inputs	Throughputs	Outputs
1._____	_____	_____
2._____	_____	_____
3._____	_____	_____
4. e.g., Salaries	e.g., Decision making	e.g., Travel abroad

Agency Inputs	Throughputs	Outputs
1._____	_____	_____
2._____	_____	_____
3._____	_____	_____
4. e.g., Budget alloca- tion	e.g., Staff meeting	e.g., Counseling

Exercise 2: Communicating Our Message to Others

Based on the model of two-unit interaction, trace the flow of communication between yourself and some relevant person, group, organization in your current workload, for example, between yourself and:

- a colleague in another department,
- your child or spouse,
- your supervisor,
- some person or group in your care,
- your employer (the boss), or
- a member of some key committee.

Try to stress the systemic aspects of the relationships in your analysis. Based on the above analysis, what suggestions do you have for making your communication more effective? Is the model sufficient for your purposes? If not, what additional concepts are required?

Exercise 3: Identify the Functions

In the appropriate columns of Table 3.4, indicate what you think are the major function(s) of the indicated components of the community (system) in which you reside. Mark major functions with the number three (3), average with a two (2), minimal with a one (1), and zero (0) for none at all. Model answers are supplied for the first two lines.

TABLE 3.4. "Figuring" Out the Functions

Community Component	Systemic Functions				
	Social-ization	Partici-pation	Mutual Aid	Econ-omy	Social Control
Police	2	0	1	0	3
Blue Cross	1	0	3	3	1
Clergy					
Welfare					
High School					
City Hall					
Industry					
Alcoholics Anonymous					
Political Party					
Public TV					
NASW Chapter					
_____					
_____					

Exercise 4: Helping the D. Family

As helpers who care about the D. family's welfare, you have decided to help the family improve its throughput processes. For example:

1. Assuming you have diagnosed the cause(s) of their problems, how would you help Betty or other members of the D. family learn (i.e., experience re-socialization) that they might change their behaviors in a desired direction?

2. How would you try to alter the D. family's equilibrium with its environment so that the family does not avoid harsh realities by closing its boundary more firmly?

3. As part of your intervention, with what other systems in the nearby environment might you link the D. family? What sort of new inputs would you hope to make available to the family as a result of these linkages?

4. If your plan includes initiating some organizational changes at Betty's place of work, suggest one or two specific interventions.

Chapter 4

System Change

INTRODUCTION

Mills (1959), Lewin (1961), and many others criticize systems analysis claiming that the model's use of functions, boundaries, equilibrium, etc., strengthens the hand of people who favor the status quo. Actually, such arguments are based on a confusion of the model (the analytic tool) with reality itself. The mirroring of self-maintenance (Chetkow 1967, Parsons 1970, Zimbalist 1961), which happens to be characteristic of most urban organizations, should not be used to discredit a systems method that reveals such self-maintenance. If urban systems and environments tend toward conservatism, it would be a mistake to blame the analytic tool for the behavior which it analyzes accurately.

This chapter tries to show how systems analysis can, in fact, be utilized in order to bring about deliberate change. After the initial definitions, you will look at four basic types of change and some of the variables which lead to change outcomes. Based on concepts learned in the last two chapters, you will be able to explore how deliberate change might be initiated by intervening in a system's inputs, throughputs, outputs, functions, feedback, boundary, linkage mechanisms, and environment. Two case examples are presented to help you concretize the idea. Actually, one report of change at the organizational level is presented twice: once in a traditional format and again using systems concepts. This material will conclude by considering the implications for social work practice of a systemic way of conceptualizing change.

WHAT IS "CHANGE"?

Koheleth, son of David when he was King in Jerusalem, was convinced that change is an illusion, as stated in his well-known cadences, "that which hath been is that which shall be, and that which hath been done is that which shall be done, and there is nothing new under the sun (Ecclesiastes 1:9)." The Nobel-winning biologist Albert Szent-Gyorgi (1962) agreed that our world did not change essentially until the middle of the nineteenth century. He was amused to think that if Napoleon and Julius Caesar could meet, they could discuss all their military and political problems without difficulty. The intervening two thousand years made no difference; however, he argued, science had changed all that in the past few decades. Small wonder that President Abraham Lincoln, in his second annual message to the United States Congress in 1862, said prophetically that "the dogmas of the quiet past are inadequate to the stormy present. Let us disenthrall ourselves."

A useful definition of the concept "change" usually includes a look at the variables in the following text.

Creating Something New

The concept of change is, in itself, very complex. There is change that is the creation of something new (or a new outcome) over the passage of a unit of time (like the birth of a baby after nine months of gestation or the building of a city like Brasilia where there had been jungle only a few years before). As you may remember from Chapter 2, had the PTO of the white suburban grade school succeeded in organizing a joint educational program with a predominantly black city school, they would have created something new in their district.

Quantitative or Ordinal Differences

Change can mirror a quantitative or ordinal transition from smaller to larger or from much to little (like the child who becomes an adult, the self-help group that evolves into a social movement, or the summer resort that becomes a ghost town during the winter months). The gradual deterioration in Betty D.'s functioning (described in Chapter 3) is another example of negative ordinal change.

Shifts of Form

Other changes are shifts of form only, as when the multigenerational family norm changes into one of the nuclear family, ice melts into water, or a voluntary service association becomes a public welfare department. The changes at the recreation center, which are described at the end of this chapter, constitute an example of a shift in form at the organizational level.

Producing a Qualitative Difference

Change can also be the transformation of one compound, state, or condition into a qualitatively different one (as when the two gases hydrogen and oxygen combine explosively to form water and heat, a chronically dependent adult becomes capable of independent living, or when, according to the German philosopher Hegel, thesis and antithesis integrate into a new synthesis). The changes in the P. family (described in Chapter 2) are of this nature.

A rural village which grows, over a twelve-year period, into a regional urban-industrial center will have undergone many of the four types of change outlined above.

You may be accustomed to visualizing change in linear or one-dimensional terms (like the way one kind of microbe always causes smallpox, or chronological age is used in the measurement of potential intellectual capacity). This is particularly true of closed systems or reductionist thinking about causality. Others see change in open systems (like the transition from normal to delinquent behavior, from youth to aging, or from tribalism to nationhood) as multidimensional. Today, such open system changes as Betty D.'s deterioration or the maturation of the mother of the P. family are defined as a process of evolving through a series of interlocking stages (Goldstein 1973, Forder 1982).

SOME CONDITIONS
THAT LEAD TO SOCIAL CHANGE

In systems analysis, it becomes more and more difficult to distinguish between cause and result. In fact, every variable can function both as a cause and an outcome at different times, and a powerful impact on any one part of a system reverberates throughout the entire system.

In light of the previous discussion, we probably should look at types of conditions that lead to social change, rather than expect a neat linear picture of cause and effect. Some of these follow.

Economic Changes

Social change can be stimulated by a disruption in economic conditions (see the discussion of the production-distribution-consumption function later in this chapter). Inflation, a long economic depression, or a flood of new resources usually lead to personal, organizational, community, and even societal changes. The threat of early retirement, which may have exacerbated Betty D.'s distress, and a change-of-job opportunity which Mrs. P. found for her husband, are partial examples of this change factor. In Chapter 3, an incremental increase of operating budget at the community center helped move its process of organizational change along.

New Ways of Thinking

A second commonly recognized cause of change is the influence of some new idea or way of thinking whose time has come, i.e., when such an idea manages to penetrate the system's boundary as a new and attractive input. Checkland (1981) reviews the impact of such ideas as energy, information, and relativity on the paradigm of scientific thinking in the Western world, and how these ideas gave birth to enormous innovations in practical technology. New ideas can also lead to drastic changes in values, norms, and expectations. For example, try to recall the upheavals caused by the idea that the world was round during the era of Columbus, the idea of "freedom" throughout Africa after World War II, and that "black is beautiful" among African-American citizens of the United States during the lifetime of Martin Luther King. Modern therapy probably became possible once mental illness was conceptualized as caused behavior and not as punishment for sinful acts.

Crisis

Another condition leading to system change is crisis. This is often precipitated by an overload of inputs (or demands) from the system's environment or by a sudden spurt of internal systemic growth. Think of the changes brought about by the extra demands of a population explosion, a disastrous flood, a factory closing in a small town, or learning that one has cancer. Crisis can also lead to outcomes such as creative problem solving and personal growth, as in the case of Mrs. P.

Prigogine and Stengers (1984) argue that, in open systems, the instability of a crisis condition makes radical choice making necessary. When such decisions cannot be avoided, they lead to outcomes which spread rapidly throughout the system and may bring about a new steady state. For example, a 1973 political crisis in Israel gave birth to an angry citizen protest movement which grew into a popular political party. It was so successful in the next elections that it received two cabinet posts and became part of the governing power coalition it had recently opposed. The suddenness of this rise to a position of power led to an intense struggle for control among its leaders (i.e., a serious crisis). Soon afterward, the party was coopted by the establishment, and rendered ineffective—all of the above happening within a period of four years.

Leaders

Taylor (1975) and others stress the part of influential leaders in bringing about major social changes. Such leaders seem to stimulate traditional throughputting in radical new ways. Certainly, the increasing openness in Russia during the late 1980s was a product of the leadership of Mikhail Gorbachev. Similarly, the excitement of the early years of America's great society was connected to the personality of President John Kennedy and the political skills of Lyndon Johnson who followed him. Mrs. P.'s leadership skills helped rally her family, whereas the lack of clear leadership in Betty D.'s family seemed to intensify the suffering of all its members. We might well remember the significant changes brought about by talented evil leaders such as Adolf Hitler.

Your knowledge of systems ideas should have alerted you to the possibility that many change-stimulating factors may themselves be the outcome of other or previous changes. For example, few would dispute that innovations in communication have eliminated distances and encouraged cosmopolitanism, or that the technology of printing invented by Gutenberg led to a significant increase in literacy. When the steam locomotive replaced the horse around the middle of the nineteenth century, the Western world entered a new era. Another era was ushered in by the spread of electronic and computer technology. However, did these factors cause urbanization (or the value revolution called modernization), were they correlated with urbanization, or were they the results of gradual urbanization? According to reductionist thinking, results come after causes. In the systems paradigm, causes become contributing variables as either inputs or components. Each one is affected by change in the functioning of any one of the others.

CHANGE IN SYSTEMIC TERMS

System analysts look at change with a range of tools and axioms. In systems terms, change can show in many ways, such as inputs-throughputs-outputs, feedback, boundary, intersystemic linkages, systemic functions, and environmental changes.

Inputs-Throughputs-Outputs

Capelle (1979) suggests that systemwide changes will follow alterations of inputs (e.g., the P. family's new contacts with various social agencies, an industry's access to additional budget, and governmental pressures to hire certain kinds of people), alterations in throughputs (e.g., formal or informal decision making or internal allocations of available human resources), or alterations of outputs (e.g., products/services wanted or rejected by other systems in the environment and Mr. P.'s work as a mailman). In summary, if a baby (the system) gets a balanced diet, is cared for by relatively calm and loving adults, and is appreciated by grandparents and family friends (inputs), his/her metabolism will make for normal growth (throughput) to create behaviors (outputs) such as health, smiles, creativity, and cooperation. Such a child is not likely to become a chronic bed wetter.

Feedback

Systems may change if their feedback processes are disturbed. For example, accurate economic or demographic data from market research helps large industries produce consumer goods the public will buy and avoid investing in products that cannot be marketed. Misreading or overlooking such feedback can lead to bankruptcy. Similarly, university students who receive critiques of classroom performance or grades for written assignments see themselves on closed-circuit video, are praised for creative risk taking (forms of feedback), learn rapidly and with high levels of satisfaction. Agency clients (like Mrs. P. and her older children) required positive and negative feedback from their social worker and significant others in their everyday lives in order to progress from chronic dependency to a basic level of self-reliance.

Boundary

Helping a system's boundary to become more open or more closed is another way to bring about change. When an urban renewal agency adds local residents to its steering committee (i.e., when the boundary is opened up), the agency's operational priorities are very likely to change (Skynner 1974). On the other hand, closing ranks against talented but nonconformist staff persons can so isolate them that their abilities to intervene effectively are negated. Similarly, inmates from open prisons who undergo gradual rehabilitation (i.e., the boundary of their system is made flexible before they are released) are less likely to return after a few months than are those released unprepared from a maximum-security prison. During systemwide disasters, when special conditions make strong personal defenses temporarily inoperative (the boundary is opened up), social workers have unique opportunities for emergency intervention with their clients.

Intersystemic Linkages

An open boundary also makes possible the linking of systems, so that one actor functioning in two systems can create change through new relationships. In the P. family case, the social worker first linked the family with the local welfare office to guarantee the finances for a deafness therapist, and then linked the daughter with a deafness counselor. Analogous outcomes can be achieved by deliberately breaking links between systems. If a counselor advised Betty D. to leave her job or divorce her husband, such de-linkages would certainly lead to change. The success of a probation officer's work often depends on separating a released prisoner from former neighborhood buddies.

Loomis (1959 and 1975) suggests ways to achieve specific or directed social change by means of systemic linkage. According to him, most change agents (people responsible for implementing a project's goals in a professional way, like the consultant in the settlement house story at the end of this chapter) usually begin work from outside the system that is to be changed. They engage in a variety of professional activities in order to become a legitimate part of a target system's regular functioning. In doing this, elements of diverse systems begin to function as a unitary—or linked—larger system. Of course, change agents can achieve similar results when they are part of the target system from the beginning (see Lippitt, Watson, and Westley, 1958, Warren 1971, or Pincus and Minahan 1973).

The clinic social worker in the P. case, like all Loomis-style change agents, must demonstrate that she can be relied upon for personal performance, which includes giving emotional support, and access to environmental resources. Once linked to the horizontal dynamics of the target system, these agents can exert pressure on local charismatic leaders or threaten to deny future resources in order to push the system toward desired changes. For example, Doig (1968) reports how a small voluntary (social action) organization was able to influence the New York City police to change bail and summons-issuing practices. The organization offered the police high-prestige, short-term consultation; opportunities to validate the effectiveness of the recommended new procedures; training programs; and long-term support relationships—all financed by the change sponsors themselves. The police found such an offer difficult to turn down, became linked, and changed their bail practices.

Systemic Functions

Shifting the functioning of the system's internal components can also lead to change. The alteration of the production-consumption function from private enterprise to nonmarket approaches, as in subsidies or Social Security, ushered in the era of the welfare state. In this case, a new idea—that the economy should not only take care of production and consumption but should also serve the function of mutual support—led to a widespread change of expectations (Rittel and Webber 1973, Anner 1982).

Environmental Changes

To complete the circle, changes in the environment can lead to changes in a local system, as when legislation or governmental regulations require city government, private clubs, public services, etc., to serve black customers as well as white ones. Such tactics make governmental resources available in a new way, forcing organizations which desire these inputs to adapt to new rules of the game. For social activists who want to cause critical systemic changes, Forder (1982) recommends implementing a number of power and policy changes in the environment. Among them are decentralization (as was done with Bell Telephone Company), changing the existing power base (as a result of registering new voters), or increasing centralization (as in federated fund raising).

Carl Rogers (1978) suggested that open systems display a clear-cut tendency (observed in crystals, microorganisms, organic life, and human beings) toward increasing order, interrelatedness, and complexity (Ansbacher 1978). Along with Adler, Capra, Erikson, Jantsch, Maslow, Menninger, Prigogine and Stengers, Rogers opposes an indiscriminate application of the laws of thermodynamics to open systems.

One of these laws claims that systems tend eventually to deteriorate or become disorganized (entropy). Today, scholars grant that the latter principle may be applicable to closed systems, but that the reverse seems true of open systems. Since open systems constantly seek out additional resources from their environment, they tend toward greater orderliness and complexity as they grow into maturity. This is as characteristic of a healthy child growing toward puberty as it is of networks of main and branch banks or of homes for the aged—all seeking additional inputs/resources in order to expand.

CHANGE VERSUS PROGRESS

Although all progress is a form of change, change may not always be progress. Demographic shifts (e.g., the rise of a region's number of aged persons by 10 percent in a five-year period) can be measured objectively and be described objectively. However, deciding whether this change is progress or the advent of new problems depends on the value orientation of the person who is responding. A politician, looking for an easy block of voters, might see such a development as very desirable. However, the head of the Bureau of the Budget, bearing in mind that retirees pay less taxes and are likely to require a significant increase of expensive medical and social services, may see this as a deplorable development.

Put simply, change is something that can be measured and is relatively easy to prove. If the number of people killed in car accidents rose by ten during the past year, this is part of the facts of urban life. However, if you are the parent of a child run over by a careless driver, you may well ask "when will this slaughter on the roads stop?" Our values and judgments are involved when we become convinced that some particular change is progress. It may well depend on who you ask whether urban-industrial-electronic changes are the harbingers of progress or disaster.

SYSTEM CHANGE AT THE PERSONAL LEVEL

In a one-person system, one form of change is the death of a parent, as has been described by Cho et al. (1982). These authors analyze how an adolescent might cope with death and grief by denying death rather than accepting it as part of the life cycle. Sophisticated attention to such a denial of change would include the encouragement of grieving in a supportive environment. In cases when relations with the deceased were hostile, help in overcoming guilt may be equally important. Long-range treatment might provide opportunities for grieving adolescents to learn about death and dying (socialization). They might also be helped by a peer group experience of volunteering (within the participation function) in a hospice for terminally ill people.

Cho's analysis gradually moves from helping a grief-stricken person-system to cope with the changed situation to focusing on the many environmental support systems which must be activated on behalf of young mourners (see Figure 4.1). For optimal results with grieving young persons, in their family or participatory environments, multilevel intervention might include individual or group counseling, sibling and family therapy, linkage to support from peers and other informal community networks, insurance settlements from formal community resources, and investment in environment-wide primary prevention through such socialization efforts as creating an acceptance of grieving as normative behavior. These were all to be done by caseworkers.

In general, the literature of therapy relies increasingly on system approaches. For example, Mishne argues that systems concepts would help apply ego psychology perspectives to social work practice, Compher discusses parent-school-child problems in systems terms, and Green reviews the systems orientation of family therapists—all in

FIGURE 4.1. Coping with Grief on Many Levels

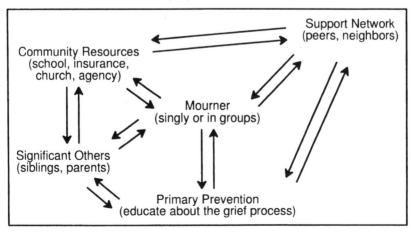

Source: Adapted from Cho et al., 1982.

volume 63 of *Social Casework* (1982). Two years earlier, Kepner (1980) insisted that gestalt therapists always operate with a systems perspective and consider therapy as a process which takes place within the boundaries of small (group) systems. According to gestalt therapy, personal growth results from healthy contact between self and the environment. Weick (1981) discusses person-in-environment in similar terms. Like Germain (1973) or Miller (1988), Weick insists that we broaden our shriveled conception of environment, giving up our body-mind dichotomy arguments to understanding human behavior and change. Climate, physical buildings, food sources, external challenges and stimulants—all are essential for normal human-social survival and growth.

SYSTEM CHANGE
AT THE ORGANIZATIONAL LEVEL

The following case illustration focuses on a service organization and is rather lengthy. Please be patient, since it first tells the story in the format of a traditional consultant's report, and then reanalyzes the same events in systems terminology. By doing Exercises 1 and 2, you should be able to apply these learnings to both macro and micro types of social work practice.

The Agency and Its Problems

The agency this story describes was founded seventeen years ago by a religious philanthropist who wanted to "offer healthy recreation programs to underprivileged children."* The Center had become a multifunctional private agency with an executive director and six professional staff members. The Center Director and the Athletics Director, who came into the field "before the university degree became so fashionable," ran the agency like their private empire (i.e., like a semiclosed system). The Center had a large operating budget, and a new gymnasium was recently donated to its

---

*Elements of this case history have been pieced together from five actual organizational reports about change efforts in Israel, Canada, and the United States.

physical plant by the family of the now-deceased founder. Its utilization statistics added up to impressive monthly totals.

Consultants from the metropolitan Federation of Neighborhood Centers were actually unhappy with this Center's style of operation. They were concerned about the large turnover each year among the volunteers, club leaders, and membership. At conferences, staff members admitted that the Center attracted middle-class users from all parts of the city, who paid for expensive activities like ceramics, while the youth of the immediate neighborhood remained untouched by the Center's programs. The Athletics Director, who loved to sponsor competitive sports which attract large audiences, was a local boy whose uncle was a member of the City Council. He and the Director were clearly proud of "their" Center's record for earning money.

Early in 1978, the Federation obtained a special grant in order to invite a faculty person from the nearby State University to help this Center change its focus—specifically to expand the services it offered to the lower-class residents of its area. For example, special funds were available for the development of a local marriage counseling service appropriate for the population of an impoverished neighborhood. With the grudging consent of the Director, the consultant was employed for a period of twenty-four months. At the end of this period, he wrote the following report, which has also been rewritten in systems terms below.

Excerpts from the Consultant's Report

During the past two years, I worked with the Center's Board of Directors and staff in small groups and as total units. Administrative personnel, professional staff, paraprofessionals, and volunteers were involved in problem identification as well as exposure to a variety of formal and informal educational experiences. Efforts were made to introduce such innovations as a nursery school, a family counseling clinic, and day care for the aged.

From the beginning, I tried to work with the anxieties of agency personnel in small group sessions, encouraging them to trust me and to trust each other. At staff meetings, everyone was invited to participate actively in gathering data about what they do, as well as in program planning.

I began with what I thought was a positive, open relationship with the Director. However, his continuing lack of cooperation made it clear that political and economic pressures would be necessary in order to cause him to change his habits. I therefore recruited a political science colleague to exert influence within City Council and identified significant financial incentives, from the Federation's grant, in order to get the Director to stop opposing the new developments. I tried to work with the Director, specifically about his underlying opposition, sensing that he was insecure about his lack of formal education and loss of control over "his Center." I was met with smiles and denials on his part. . . .

The staff of a new subsystem within the Center, the family counseling clinic (housed, incidentally, in a nearby building), showed readiness to adopt a more neighborhood-oriented style of work. Clinical counseling gradually expanded to include working with clients in groups (e.g., single parents). In addition, family-clinic staff agreed to map their clients' addresses. They were struck by the fact that whole subareas of the neighborhood were not being served at all and decided to do some selective outreach into one of them. Over the months, I helped them hold an open house for other community professionals, make an attractive annual report (which brought their story before community influentials), advertise on the bulletin boards of targeted supermarkets, and develop a group of local volunteers. They were even able to offer a course of family-life education in the nearby high school. . . .

I often worked through others in what has been called the two-step flow of communication. This required intensive development with the Center's administrative and program department heads until they felt ready to accept some additional (neighborhood) responsibilities, and then to convince their workers and volunteers to go along. I wanted to bring them to a condition of shared responsibility rather than let them become dependent on some expert to make decisions for them (Katz 1963).

I also tried to strengthen interagency working relations in the metropolitan community. After some eighteen months of process, the Center invited representatives of five other local agencies and City Hall to a public meeting. I gave a short talk on the dynamics of cooperative efforts, and led the discussion of issues that followed. The meeting ended with many agency persons expressing a willingness to go on. However, the Center Director, whose opposition had been passive all this time, was so threatened by the prospect of having to cooperate with other community institutions that he found excuses for not convening the forum again. Had this effort continued beyond the initial meeting, we could have created a local interagency council (Baker, Broskowski, and Brandwein 1973, Mott 1968). Alas, the Director sabotaged that. . . .

Two years later, I learned that the Director had left the Center for employment in a commercial recreation service. We are still polite to each other professionally, but he seems to be avoiding me at meetings.

A SYSTEMS ANALYSIS
OF ORGANIZATIONAL CHANGE

If the consultant in the previous example had been a systems analyst, he would have described his interventions in terminology more like the summaries at the end of Chapters 2 and 3. No doubt the language used below is different from that of the consultant's traditional prose, but you are asked to judge whether or not the systems version of his report is more precise and offers clearer options for planful intervention. The exercises at the end of this chapter should enable you to use this type of systems analysis on any episode within your current practice.

A New Paradigm for Looking at Organizations

Most of us tend to think of public or social services as large bureaucratic organizations, and such organizations are usually pictured as pyramids. Of course, an executive director or chief executive officer functions at the top of the pyramid, and power arrangements are hierarchial. It is equally useful to reconceptualize such organizations in terms of circles (see Figure 4.2). Now the central executive person becomes a coordinator or focalizer, and the reality of horizontal and vertical relations is much more obvious. Power now becomes something shared by short-term coalitions. The role of the consultants as bridges to resources in the environment (future agency inputs) is also clear.

FIGURE 4.2. A Nonbureaucratic Organizational Picture of the Center

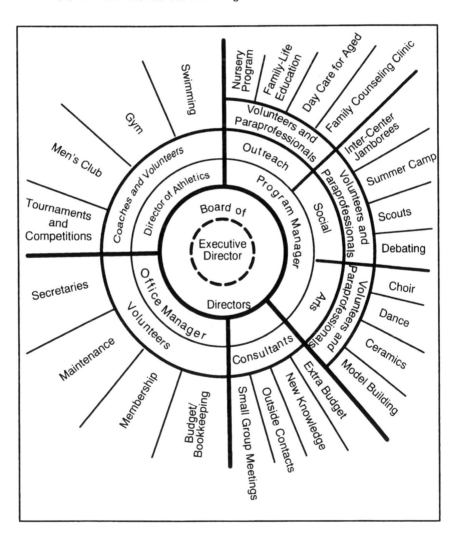

Environment

People from impoverished neighborhoods can be seen as having spent their formative years in a dull or barren environment, as being stigmatized as "welfare parasites," and as feeling abandoned within this closed neighborhood setting.

If the Center is defined as the system, its environment contains the City Council, other social agencies, the municipality/community, other nearby towns, regional and national offices of various social services, the Ministry of Welfare, the Treasury, etc. The practice of using circular organizational diagrams can also be used to elaborate the Center's relationships with such service or political organizations in its environment (shown in Figure 4.3). A bureaucratic Center director would very likely find the prospect of sharing power with so many of his neighbors very threatening. He resisted the idea throughout the episode.

Change might have been initiated by means of critical news media reports, protests by well-organized welfare rights groups, an ombudsman, or a public service lawsuit. In this case, the Federation chose to use the social control approach of offering financial and prestige incentives for accepting the consultant (change agent) within the system. Political power was also activated in the Center's environment in order to get Center staff working on the needs of the local neighborhood.

Boundary, Steady State, Inputs

As discussed above, deliberate strategies were used by the consultant-intervener to open up the formerly closed boundaries of the Center's top staff. The opened-up boundary made possible many new vertical inputs such as budget changes, paraprofessional and volunteer personnel, support from other agencies and funding bodies, etc.

After the system became sensitized to its poverty neighborhood environment, it also became open to the possibility of equilibrium disturbance. Gradually, the Center's boundary condition changed from that of equilibrium to one more like steady state.

The latter made possible a two-way flow (or exchange) of inputs and outputs, which the Center staff found enriching.

FIGURE 4.3. Relationships Between the Center and Other Systems in Its Environment

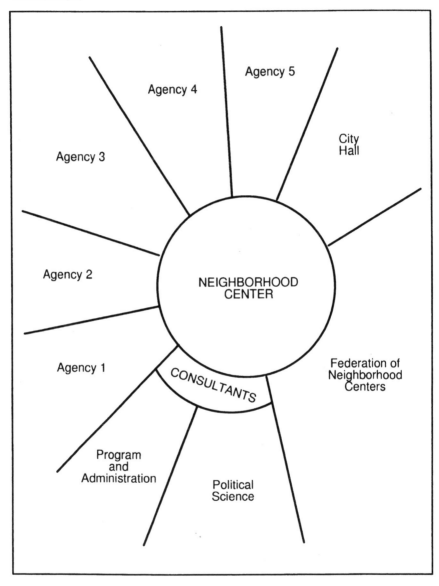

Linkages

It was necessary to weaken the strong link that the Director and the Head of Athletics had to the local power structure in order to make program changes possible at the Center. Relevant interventions were therefore mounted in the environment.

Board members and personnel, separately and together, discovered that they were linked with neighborhood systems and with other service agencies in the community. Working in new partnerships with such systems and subsystems, the Center's focus of operations gradually broadened.

Output

Former Center outputs of recreation services for middle-class users continued, although in lessening quantities, over the two-year consultation period.

New outputs (e.g., through the marital counseling clinic) were initiated and sustained.

Although the Center's professional staff had always kept in contact with other social service agencies in the community, there was a noticeable increase in referral of Center clients to other agencies in the region. Center staff persons also found themselves in demand as consultants to other agencies, after they felt secure in serving a lower-class population.

Functions and Throughput

Attractive development workshops, training programs, and short courses were made available, and Center staff were encouraged to try some of the new learnings and skills within their regular workloads. In this process of resocialization, the consultant served as expert, teacher, and role model in order to help change former throughput patterns.

Despite the unenthusiastic backing of the Center Director, sanctions and rewards (social control) were altered as soon as the new approach proved acceptable to the majority of the Center's Board. Particular effort was invested in expanding available staff rewards, including praise, time off, recognition through promotions, salary increases, and readiness to give staff a measure of autonomy to experiment with new programs.

The participation function was changed drastically, resulting in many new forms of throughput. Department heads were invited to participate in Board meetings and serve as experts in meetings of subcommittees. Staff meetings changed from the passive reception of instructions to worker-initiated study sessions and data-gathering efforts. One neighborhood resident, a known leader, was added to each subcommittee, and their contributions gradually led to a shift in programmatic emphases.

The increase of economic resources for the Center generally, and for its poverty-related new programs specifically, needs no elaboration. The additional inputs of public support proved a pleasant surprise to the agency Director. With increased resources, the Center's volume and range of outputs also expanded.

Feedback

The increase in staff participation also generated a willingness to improve the accountability and recording (feedback to the community) procedures of all personnel. The staff also seemed ready for group self-evaluation.

Once residents became part of the Center's committee process, an improvement was noted in the quality of feedback from the field concerning output effectiveness.

Coherence

At the start of the organizational process, Center staff themselves showed varying degrees of anxiety and resisted the consultant's proposed changes. The Director, for instance, tried to avoid getting involved (perhaps from fear of losing his authority or control of "his" agency), in spite of the consultant's efforts to open communications with him. Perhaps, if the same consultant had involved a colleague— from the Psychology or Social Work Department of the university— ways might have been found to cope with the Director's fears and lack of trust. The change process might have produced more results (outputs) if the Director had been able to make him into a full partner.

Nevertheless, other consultant inputs did lead to the Center staff themselves noticing a rise in morale. They showed a parallel increase in willingness to invest extra time and effort in the work. Formal rituals of cooperation and sharing became more natural. Rewards (such as praise from the consultant or expressed interest from a Board member) became effective instruments of positive reinforcement, as did repeated, spontaneous gifts of home baking from residents later in the change process.

The consultant noted a difference in how staff talked about their work. Criticism and complaining decreased slowly, and a tendency to accentuate the positive could be detected.

SUMMARY

The above analytic model should apply equally effectively to other types of organizations (e.g., a Public Welfare office, a Family Service Association, a United Fund campaign). As you know, systems analysis does not lay out a mechanical structure or anatomy. On the contrary, systems models help show a piece of reality in all its dynamic complexity. Because of the interdependence of component parts within a system, changing one component tends to reverberate throughout the entire system. If a system component is also linked vertically to a unit within another system, change in one system is likely to be accompanied by change in the linked partner. Finally, if a system's inputs exceed its outputs, persons/groups/organizations will go through a succession of normal life cycle changes, fulfilling functions essential for survival and growth.

At this point, you should be able to analyze change in a systems way. After looking at some conditions conducive to change in many kinds of systems, you learned that change usually comes about in nonlinear ways, and explored a range of systems situations that stimulate change.

In short, a systems approach should help you comprehend the multiple causes of a continuing problem condition. It also provides some hints as to effective channels through which deliberate change might be begun and then sustained. This topic is elaborated on in the next chapter.

EXERCISES

Exercise 1: Identifying Conditions That Lead to Change

With full appreciation of the complexity of cause-finding in systems analysis and with reference to the materials just presented, describe one real-life example of change and of some of the causes of this outcome. Use examples that led to significant changes in your professional practice or in your day-to-day life (see Table 4.1). In your example, are there instances of multicausality? If so, describe this situation in one or two short paragraphs, and indicate what special type of change resulted from these causes occurring together as they did.

TABLE 4.1. Finding the Components of Change

"Causes" (Inputs)	Change (Outcomes)
Economics:_____	_____
_____	_____
New Ideas:_____	_____
_____	_____
Crisis:_____	_____
_____	_____
Leader(s):_____	_____
_____	_____
Other(s):_____	_____
_____	_____

Exercise 2: Analyzing Deliberate Systemic Change

Focusing on the concepts listed below, try using them to look again at the P. family story, or at an episode in your caseload:

- Environment
- Boundary
- Steady State
- Inputs
- Linkages

- Outputs
- Functions
- Throughput
- Feedback
- Coherence

Chapter 5

Systems Analysis
of Some Social Work Practices

INTRODUCTION

One useful feature of the systems model is its capacity to identify the many levels involved in any open system problem (Fuller 1977, Kasarda 1974). The model also helps clarify the fact that social work interventions are undertaken to prevent problems from developing, or to rehabilitate those who are caught up in a problem (see discussion later in this chapter).

A detailed history of the evolution of systems thinking in social work literature is found in Appendix A. At this point, you should remember the pioneer work of Lippitt and his associates in 1958, the relative silence of the 1960s, and the outpouring of interest which followed. In one decade, system-related materials were published by Germain, Goldstein, Kahn, Pincus and Minahan, Hearn, and Siporin. These social work scholars agreed on the desirability of developing a unitary (clinical-social-environmental) model of social work practice. A systems-based approach was seen as being able to free the profession from its over-reliance on both practice methods and the medical model of healing sickness—concepts which were still popular twenty years after the publication (Chin 1961) of *The Planning of Change*. The evolving systems model was perceived to be equally applicable to fields of practice, service delivery, policy, and administration (Bleodorn et al. 1977, Germain 1973 and 1978).

This chapter is designed to help you apply systems analysis to the definitions of needs, problems, clients, and targets. Intervention activities are analyzed as five-stage episodes. Appropriate professional roles are suggested for each stage, and all are illustrated with practice examples.

DEFINING PROBLEMS AND NEEDS SYSTEMICALLY

Rittel and Webber (1973) claim that the reductionist paradigms of engineers do not fit problems of open systems. Since human beings develop and exist with other people in open systems, social problems are inherently different from what the authors call the "tame" problems of closed systems. You will discover, especially if you do Exercise 1, that open system problems can be very messy. Even if you can analyze them with some accuracy, they are difficult to eliminate.

Specifically in connection with open system difficulties, Rittel and Webber say the following:

1. A precise (quantitative or reductionist) formulation of the problem is seldom possible.
2. Every problem is, in large part, unique and is not particularly clarified as a result of analysis into smaller component parts.
3. Every problem can be the symptom, or the result, of another problem.
4. A situation can be explained in a number of ways: i.e., each way of analyzing the situation is as much determined by the problem solver's choices as by the nature of the problem itself.
5. Solutions are often a one-time activity, and sometimes "any" solution is satisfactory (see also Duhl 1969).
6. Solutions, or perhaps resolutions, are judged effective or ineffective in a very pragmatic sense.
7. Those responsible often have to stop, not because the problem was solved, but rather because they ran out of time, patience, money, or public support.

Social work interveners are often satisfied if they can improve some aspect of human functioning in the real world. You may have to devote effort to work on the same problem again in a few years, because open systems and their environments keep changing.

In broad systemic terms, a social problem is a way of indicating a dysfunctional or incomplete (systemic or environmental) situation which, at some point in time, requires special effort on our part to complete, or resolve. Problem situations can also be analyzed as outcomes of deviant or inadequate systemic functioning as:

1. Unmet needs are the result of input deprivation (as in the story of the P. family);
2. Blocked or distorted feedback (e.g., inadequate biological or emotional inputs, which might produce paranoia);
3. Agencies not cooperating on a common issue due to hardening of their systemic boundaries or inadequate linkage (as in the story of the white and black school systems);
4. Identity problems which result from failure to learn norms and expectations during socialization (Ackoff 1974);
5. Urban poverty which can be traced to slum residents' lack of opportunity to participate in determining the policies for the services set up to meet their needs; or
6. Barren environments so lacking in stimuli or challenges (i.e., lack of inputs) that normal systemic growth is rare or impossible.

The type of analysis/diagnosis made possible by using systemic models seems essential for effective problem resolution in the human services.

SYSTEMIC MODELS OF HUMAN DEVELOPMENT AND BEHAVIOR

Practitioners from the helping professions, like their colleagues from the social sciences, have created many models to explain patterns of human development or of types of behavior. Although they do not show a specific appreciation of systems, if we look carefully at Freud's id-ego-superego model (or at those of Piaget, Maslow, Etzioni, Warren, or Kübler-Ross), we find that these models are in fact systems-based. Some of the models are linear or sequential in format—strongly implying that the realizing of one stage is predicated on the completion of the previous one. For example, in a model geared to differences of age, work is followed by retirement after a certain birthday. Similarly, a successful grandparenthood comes after the parenthood phase. Other models focus on patterns which are nonlinear (Germain 1987). In them, the variables depend on their interlocking functions and reciprocal relationships, as illustrated by the four components of all conflicts in Chapter 6. One example of each type is presented below.

From Prevention to Damaging Sickness

A categorization of five types of social services may be presented in the format of a linear or sequential model.

1. Logically, the first type focuses on strengthening basic social institutions (e.g., the family). Called primary prevention in public health, this effort centers around enhancing normal growth (or health) by means of well-baby clinics, working for a wholesome environment (from which to receive vital inputs), and/or providing budget for sound social services. Accordingly, we send children to summer camp or encourage them to join the Boy/Girl Scouts for a healthy socialization experience. Such experiences are considered vital for their normal development as well as life-enriching. Success means the ability to prevent certain dysfunctions altogether.
2. When genetic or environmental factors are known to cause specific dysfunctions (note that in systems analysis, the idea of pathologies is abandoned), we engage in secondary prevention. Now we try to prevent the action of specific causal factors—we vaccinate against measles, improve sanitation (especially making certain that our drinking water is pure), arrange hot breakfasts in city-center (poverty-area) schools, and we may lobby for desirable new legislation. Our intention is always to accomplish the ounce of prevention which nips problems in the bud and enables all of us to live normal lives.
3. When malfunctions have, nevertheless, started and symptoms of some social-medical dysfunction (e.g., the crisis after a loved one dies, when members of a cultural minority are suddenly the targets of vicious victimization, or when children are caught selling hard drugs), we first try for immediate diagnosis and treatment. Wartime crises are processed by means of a telephone hot line. The intention is to shorten the period of suffering, to reduce the possibility of the condition worsening,

and to restore people to normal functioning as soon as possible, just as early diagnosis can catch a cancerous skin growth before the body succumbs to a full-scale traumatic illness. Prevention and crisis intervention are, of course, much less expensive per capita than having to cure and rehabilitate sick persons or to restore the functioning of an organization which has gone bankrupt.

4. If earlier intervention was impossible, and people have become seriously ill or handicapped, efforts will be made to reduce the damage, restore mobility and motivation, and (wherever possible) rehabilitate clients to an accepted level of normal living. We improvise artificial limbs for those who need them, provide wheelchairs for those who become permanently handicapped, provide counseling for unwed mothers, and help angry people experience catharsis—in order that they eventually cease to be dependent, overcome despair, and get back to the business of living well in their community.

5. When the final damage is irreversible (e.g., a retiree contracts Alzheimer's disease), we try to adapt to the situation. We minimize the chance of any side effects, and try to make the person's daily existence (often in custodial care) as comfortable as possible. We also work with the client's relatives—to help ease their pain or to help them communicate with their bedridden loved one.

The above is an example of a linear systemic model. Clearly, we hope to invest the most resources in prevention, but must be ready to supply the other four types of service in a proper sequence. When, for example, crisis intervention services do not exist in some community, the slightly ill may become critically ill and require more expensive rehabilitative and accommodation services.

Erikson's Model Ages and Stages

Back in 1950, while demonstrating how personality was linked to societal realities, Erikson proposed his now famous model of the eight stages of human development. His text suggests that these stages usually take place in an age-related sequence from childhood to grandparenthood, and his model is pictured as looking very linear.

However, Erikson himself writes that after the first (developing trust) stage, human development is not rigidly hierarchical. Stages often get skipped, without interfering with any seeming order or sequence.

Figure 5.1 suggests how Erikson's model can be visualized as eight overlapping circles. In such a reconceptualization, we deal with an eight-variable system, in which each variable influences all the other seven and is influenced by them in turn (this figure represents 56 possible interrelationships).

FIGURE 5.1. Erikson's Eight Stages of Human Development

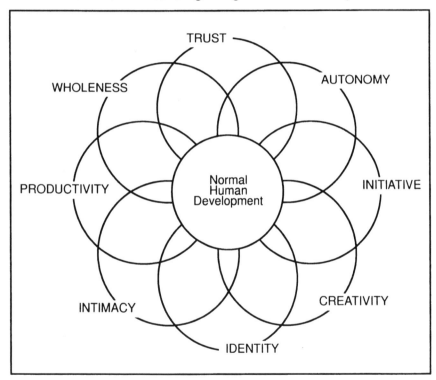

CREATING A NEW AGENCY: A CASE REPORT

The following episode of planned change took place several years ago in a city of about 200,000 people. In the initial environment all the social agencies had expressed uneasiness about the rising incidence of divorce. At a meeting of colleagues, a local family court judge related how helpless he felt one morning when a young man, in the process of a "messy" divorce, began to weep in his courtroom. His uneasiness fell on sympathetic ears and received wide media coverage.

Within weeks, citywide interest in lessening the divorce rate became operational under the auspices of the Council of Churches. By the end of the year, a well-known expert on family courts was invited to town for a week of meetings with legal, religious, and social service professionals.

Six months after these meetings, interest had grown and a *client system* began to form. A small group of lawyers, social workers, and clergymen formed a Committee of Concerned Citizens. One year later, the group was asked to become an ad hoc Task Force of the Council of Churches. The group did so, expanding its representation. It studied both the facts and skills necessary for changing the functioning of divorce courts and began to plan a court-related marriage counseling demonstration program.

Two and a half years after the initial community meeting, the project became the Domestic Relations Task Force of the Church Council; that is, the project's *action system* was formally recognized. This Task Force, which included most members of the original client system, expanded again to a total of twenty-eight active persons. Within months, five subcommittees met a total of fifteen times; the overall Committee met five times; documents were prepared; four community-wide mailings were sent out; and a two-day institute was planned. At the latter, over 100 interested citizens heard a stirring speech about court-operated domestic counseling services and responded with enthusiasm. Press coverage was generous and positive.

In the implementation stage, the expanded action system functioned at a hectic pace. Within the next three months, four new subcommittees met a total of ten times. A formal incorporation proposal was revised five times, and a budget for a three-year demonstration was worked out. Meetings were held with all local judges and with the Bar Association. Candidates were nominated for a new board of directors for a court-related counseling service.

Funding was obtained and part-time counselors were recruited. During a sixty-day compulsory waiting period (after first application to the court), couples seeking divorce were referred to the counseling service "for at least one session." All this was accomplished during the fourth of a four-year community change episode.

Eventually, the Domestic Relations Task Force gave birth to the new, highly coherent agency. After a few weeks, the new agency was offering counseling interviews in connection with all divorces handled by the courts. Before the end of the three-year demonstration period, this service became part of the court's regular functioning and its budget was incorporated into the municipal tax system. Despite subsequent efforts by the Church Council to find new projects for its Domestic Relations Task Force, meeting attendance dwindled to two or three people. The committee was eventually deactivated.

CLIENT, ACTION, AND TARGET SYSTEMS

Over the past twenty years, many scholars have stressed the important contribution of systems thinking to differentiating between client, action, and target systems (Lippitt, Watson, Westley 1958, Warren 1969 and 1971, Brager 1968, Rothman 1970, Pincus and Minahan 1973, Siporin 1975, Forder 1982).

Client System

This refers to those individuals, groups, or organizations (i.e., systems of any size) that are recognized as having the normative legitimacy to request or demand that attention (in the form of welfare-related services or service changes) be focused on a problem within a given environment. This client system usually includes the future beneficiaries of the change, staff persons from various agencies, and members of the power structure. In the same sense that the lawyer's client is responsible for setting action goals, a client system creates policy for the welfare community generally, or sets goals for its own process of learning better ways to cope. When the worker of the mental health clinic decided to send the P. family's deaf daughter to a therapist, the daughter herself was not part of a client system. Had the daughter sought help from this therapist, the client (beneficiary) and the target (defined below) systems would have become identical.

In general, the size or components of any client system can be enlarged or reduced during the change process as required by the process itself. For example, if a client system wants to locate a hallway house for slightly retarded children in a residential neighborhood, it would do well to include representatives of City Hall (for legitimacy), some relatives of potential service users (who know the needs), some technical experts or agency employees (who are essential for implementation), and representatives of the neighbors (who might, in fear, close ranks and shut the service down). In specific situations, some members of the client system may not benefit directly from the changes they help to bring about. A really effective client system will even invite members of a relevant target system (defined below) to participate in goal-setting in order to minimize resistance and prevent conflict in later stages of the project.

In the above story of the creation of a new agency, the horizontal interactions among the system's diverse components were first increased (a process usually called "development."). As the project evolved, these relationships became a means for either solving the problem or realizing the goals. Once client system self-confidence was established, the group became willing to take risks within a wider and wider environment.

Since the type of participants tends to change as the action evolves, the cost (in time, effort, money, or other resources) of maintaining horizontal involvements increases as the episode continues, and the implementation stage is the most energy-expensive. Each time the system expands, deliberate inputs must be earmarked for achieving renewed commitment, bringing newcomers up to date, and keeping old-timers satisfied. Sustained communications, whether nonverbal, oral, or written, are costly. Of course, costs rise sharply if there is opposition or resistance to overcome.

Figure 5.2 attempts to clarify the relationships between a client system, its action system and its target systems, and a change agent.

FIGURE 5.2. Client, Action, and Target Systems: Interaction with Each Other and with a Change Agent

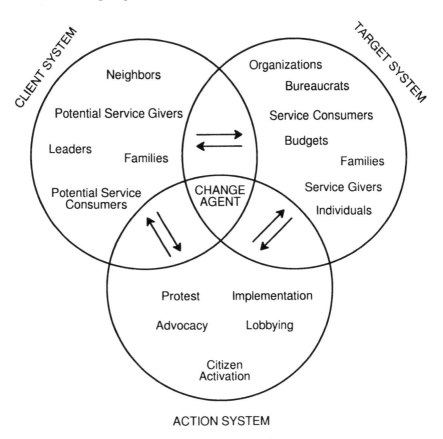

ACTION SYSTEM

Action System

This system consists of individuals, groups, or organizations (i.e., agencies or professional staff) who are capable of implementing, or of helping to implement, the client system's goals. Often this unit includes a team of workers activated or coordinated by the change agent (defined below). The action system is different from the client system in that it contains more people with technical expertise and few community notables. It may also include some target system members.

Like the client system, action systems can be of any size, in accordance with the requirements of the change process being attempted. In the story of creating new divorce services, the Council of Churches constituted the action system.

Target System

This system contains individuals, groups, or organizations whose behavior must be altered in order to implement the project goals or achieve the desired results. The targets of a change process (such as rehabilitation from a hard drug addiction) may be the beneficiaries themselves (drug addicts who ask for help in "kicking the habit"). However, many targets are clearly distinct from the client system which sets the goals. For example, an agency director (narrow client system) might employ a consultant (action system) to teach professional and administrative personnel (target system) how to cope with potentially violent drug addicts. The existing divorce courts and adversary procedures were targets of the community change process described above.

The people participating in a probationers' group are indeed the targets of an action system's therapeutic efforts, but they were sent to the group by a court order, a separate and distinct client system. In contrast, people who chose to come to a caseworker for help with their marital behavior become a unified client/target system. In a community system, policy makers, budget allocators, direct service providers, political influence holders, or coordination-planning bodies can be target systems—depending on the nature of the action goals or changes originally desired by the client system. Delineating the targets accurately, with the help of sophisticated diagnostic skills, is essential to the success of any change effort.

The Change Agent

When, in a process of deliberate change, the above three systems interact dynamically with each other, a change agent is likely to be operating behind the scenes. Even though this agent may be an employee of any of the three systems, his/her activities are unique. This person creates interaction between the three systems rather than promoting the interests of any one of them.

Change agents usually function as part of the action system. However, they also represent the entire community—sometimes having to work for change in the action system to which they belong. When they play a directive role as implementer or adminis-trator, their focus must remain community-wide.

The change agent has to have generalist skills. If anyone brings the three systems together on a project, each system also encom-passes its own complexity of components. For example, client sys-tems are oriented to individual citizens, families, neighbors, and probably local leaders. Target systems, on the other hand, focus themselves on organizations, bureaucrats, budgets, and specific ser-vices. Finally, action systems get involved in protest, advocacy, lobbying, and implementing. It takes a sophisticated change agent to activate all three of the above systems without overidentifying with any one and to help all the participants feel that their effort to achieve something together is really worthwhile.

STAGES OF THE ACTION EPISODE

In 1963, Warren postulated a five-stage systems model for ana-lyzing an "episode" of community activity. At this point, his model has been generalized in order to make it relevant to small, as well as large, systems and to suggest how client, target, and action systems interrelate.

Warren originally focused on the five stages of an episode of system change (see Figure 5.3). However, in outlining this five-phase model, he did not touch on the professional roles that a social worker might play during each phase. Appropriate role possibilities are suggested below.

1. Initial Systemic Environment

In the initial phase, a new or renewed concern is expressed regarding a specific problem-situation (e.g., an unmet need) or

FIGURE 5.3. Flowchart of a Systemic Episode

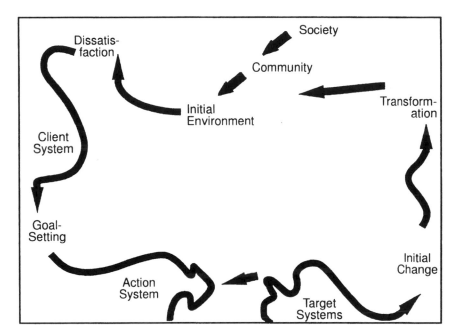

regarding a desire for something better (e.g., the above story of creating a new court-based divorce service). Earlier patterns of problem solving are examined critically, and a sense of common interest is recognized among those who care. Gradually, people of a like mind (perhaps stimulated by new leadership or by the knowledge of some technological innovation) inquire about alternative ways to tackle a problem. Shared discontent with the status quo creates expectations for change.

This is as true when a group of residents wants an improvement in neighborhood cleanliness, a teenager decides to do something about being chronically overweight, or the community leaders are upset about the residing rates of divorce). The discontent of the P. family's physician, and of Mrs. P. with young Mark's continued bed wetting led to their search for new kinds of help. Mrs. P. was also concerned about her husband's backaches and one daughter's deafness and the other's poor showing in school. Important changes emerged from her perception of this initial environment.

Appropriate Professional Role

Expressions of dissatisfaction, or of a growing desire to do something to improve a situation, often emerge during this phase without the help of a professional intervener. When such a worker is involved—as were the staff of the Federation of Neighborhood Centers who initiated the change process at the recreation center in Chapter 4—the professional role required is that of *Stimulator.*

2. Creating a Client System

In phase two, the individual or group moves from expressing dissatisfaction to collecting available facts (i.e., new inputs) and deciding what to do about the problem. They identify relevant partners in the environment (the client system) with whom to tackle the situation in a structured way. The process of choosing immediate as well as long-range goals is one of the many important throughputs. Client system members should agree about project goals; but these goals may have to be very general to make consensus possible. In any case, a person is unlikely to agree to start a diet, or a group of lower-class blacks consider seeking self-respect by participating in a consciousness raising program, unless they are really convinced that this is necessary and find support for their resolve to do something about it.

In the P. family story, Mrs. P. and her husband constitute the client system.

Appropriate Professional Role

Once the second phase has begun, the intervener (see change agent, below) functions as an *Organizer, Facilitator,* or *Guide* (Fraley 1969, Ross and Lappin 1967, Rothman 1974). By creating a process of confidence building, the intervener encourages a client system to take responsibility for setting goals regarding its members or some other target system. The clinic social worker, using well-honed powers of empathy, used similar interventions in order to help Mrs. P. and her family (in Chapter 2). In group situations, the intervener helps potential leaders take the initiative, ask questions which help clarity the problem, and/or stimulate like-minded persons to band together and seek answers. This did not take place in the case history of the white and black schools because of inadequate communication and/or feedback processes.

3. An Action System Evolves

During the third phase, plans are made concerning action priorities and relevant target systems. The circle of participants may have to be expanded in order to include persons not originally part of the client system but having talents or contacts appropriate for implementing the desired action. As soon as the person or group is ready to act, it tries to establish itself as having the solution most relevant to the issue under consideration. Moreover, above-average skills in negotiation may be essential for reaching agreement on a treatment contract or for accepting a complex interorganizational action plan. Possibilities for success are enhanced if representatives of relevant target systems have been consulted or invited to participate in this phase of the episode.

In the P. family story, the clinic social worker and the deafness therapist (both of whose outputs created new inputs for the family and caused its members to try some new kinds of throughputs) constitute the action system. Mrs. P. and all other members of her family (now the client/target system) cooperate because they were involved from the earliest phases of their episode.

Appropriate Professional Role

At this point in the episode, the client system must dare to question accepted practices and bring unfinished business to the attention of relevant actors in the system/environment. A readiness to take risks emerges only after sufficient information has been collected from expert sources. If the interveners cannot fulfill this role, they may have to import *Experts* or *Consultants* from the wider environment. As in the story of changes at the recreation center, consultants act as horizon expanders, offering a range of experiential and theoretic knowledge objectively without taking part in either previous goal determination or subsequent implementation.

Still within this phase, the expanded action system requires the intervention of an *Enabler* or *Change Agent*. The latter's ability to mediate the desires of diverse interest groups is essential. As in the case of developing a new divorce service, the enabler keeps communication channels open among system participants, as well as between system participants and important actors in their environment. This role calls for nondirective skills, working through natural leaders or committee chairpersons.

4. The Action System Implements

If enough time was allowed to accomplish the previous three phases completely, and the action (or output) phase is sustained over an appropriate period of time, you may begin to observe some changed functioning in the target systems. There will be a short-term centralization of available resources in order to enhance implementation efforts. Professional helpers, whether diet counselors or community workers, will employ human relations as well as power skills in order to bring about the changes planned in phase three.

At some point, an urban renewal neighborhood repaints buildings, plants gardens, and organizes a neighborhoodwide committee. Similarly, groups of overweight people (or oppressed African-Americans) might attend classes in consciousness-raising and form support groups. Thus, as casework treatment was provided for Mrs. P., her husband changed jobs, and a deafness counselor worked with their daughter. The action system created communitywide support for trying an experimental counseling program within the court system.

Appropriate Professional Role

During this stage, the intervener functions as a partisan *Administrator*, *Implementer*, or *Advocate*. This is an active or directive role, often demanding the efficient utilization of power to cope with resistance and bring about desired changes in a short time span. The implementer (though still empathetic) must be tough, agile, skilled in using a number of strategies simultaneously, and able to maintain inter-system links forged in the previous phase.

This worker, like the consultant who worked with the recreation center, is responsible for motivating desired changes in the behavior of relevant target systems. The recreation center consultant was, in fact, only partly successful in his role as implementer of planned change. He might have done better had he recruited some advice about empathy from social work or psychology colleagues.

5. System Transformation

As soon as the goals are close to realization, the action system tends to dissolve (e.g., the Domestic Relations Task Force of the Church Federation) or to become transformed (into a new divorce counseling service). Persons who cohered during the episode now feel free to go on vacation or devote their energies to another project. Similarly, individuals who have completed a course of therapy tend to emerge with a sense of being "a new person." A clean separation from the therapist or a graduation ceremony, along with rewards or recognition for achievement, is vital.

If the neighborhood association proves stable and is able to keep the area clean, or if an overweight teenager stays slim (i.e., finds new ways to be fulfilled), their episodes may be closed with a sense of accomplishment. Similarly, when Mark P. stops wetting his bed, Mr. and Mrs. P. quarrel less, and the younger daughter's school grades improve, transformation has begun.

Appropriate Professional Role

During transformation, the intervener should gradually withdraw. A skilled worker should find indirect ways to see that valid changes in target system behaviors are properly rewarded and that long-active members of the client/action system are recognized for their efforts.

Incidentally, sophisticated change agents should be able to fill every one of the above professional roles as appropriate to the particular phase of the episode in which they are engaged. Depending on local circumstances (for example, when an especially sensitive topic must be discussed or a vote is to be avoided), it may prove useful to import an expert from outside the system. The local intervener remains free to guide and enable, without losing the trust of either the client or the action systems.

INPUT OR BOUNDARY MANAGEMENT

Social work practitioners often help client/target persons to improve, or just change, the inputs upon which they depend for survival or growth. This may require either better information gathering about themselves and the environment, or finding and utilizing better quality resources from the environment (Weick 1981).

You may, therefore, want to focus on systemic inputs. Some authors recommend deliberate efforts to prevent dysfunctional behaviors in the first place. For example, they want to "turn off" the environmental precursors of delinquency, much in the way public health vaccinations make people independent by strengthening their bodies' resistance to the negative stimuli ever present in the environment. Relying on Lewinian field theory, you could recommend expending energy controlling the environmental factors which make people on probation return to jail. One way to do this is to harden the system's boundaries (e.g., keep a probationer away from the influence of his/her former delinquent gang and neighborhood).

Gilmore (1982) takes another approach to boundary management. He writes of the changing nature of employee-managed organizations, contending that as they decline in authoritarian leadership, they suffer from lack of clear internal boundaries between leaders and followers. Chronic frustration also accompanies this decline in clarity between non-authoritarian leaders and their increasingly independent followers.

Another aspect of input control relates to the kind of help available from the therapeutic environment. Forder (1982) indicates that a Freudian therapist will help a client/target system gain insight into the impact of the unconscious, thereby clearing the way for improving ego strengths. A caseworker like Mary Richmond (1922, 1930) would provide material resources and try to influence various power centers, such as schools and the police, on a probationer's behalf. A systems-oriented family therapist like Siporin (1975) lists both internal interventions (e.g., redefine the situation, reduce stress, refocus attention, change roles) and environmental ones (e.g., transfer to another therapeutic setting, participate in a different group, utilize various community resources). Each could generate new inputs in order to help service consumers (i.e., clients) improve their condition.

THROUGHPUT MANAGEMENT

As described in Chapter 2, throughput is the process by which a system acts upon energy, information, or raw materials (the inputs from its environment) and transforms them into internal resources and outputs. For example, advice and support from a professional social worker becomes an input for Mrs. P. (the client/target system) and enables her to alter her patterns of throughputs (to cope with stress differently or change her way of making decisions about her children). Throughput also includes the allocation (or reallocation) of existing resources in order to defend oneself effectively against system-threatening conditions, compete with a rival, etc. (Janchill 1969). The operation of free choice, or will, as well as responsibility for the consequences of such choices, is integral to all discussions of throughput.

In social work, change agents start with inputs or resources and help a target system convert them into decisions, techniques, tasks, or roles (throughputs) in order to produce changes (outputs) in individual, group, organization, or community targets. Achieving a change in patterns of throughputs is crucial to all micro and macro change efforts. For example, in relating to a delinquent neighborhood gang, the street worker first helped gang members find alternative ways for obtaining status (e.g., from helping younger kids rather than robbing old people). The satisfaction derived from this new behavior, though initially a small change, enabled some members to generalize their experiences into other areas of positive group behavior a few months later. These problem-ridden teenagers were also helped to expand their goals beyond immediate gratification toward a long-range aspiration of improved literacy and employment. Through a patient process of trust building and experiential learning, the throughputs of both the group and many of its individual members were changed irrevocably.

FEEDBACK MANAGEMENT

Feedback processes are seen as vital in all proper communication. As suggested in Figure 5.4, one thing a social worker can do to enhance the communication process is to ensure that both the sender and the receiver give the same meanings to words/symbols in their messages. For example, in a situation of ongoing tension between husband and wife, it is often essential to help both parties review what one of them (the sender) actually tried to say or to clarify that what the spouse (the receiver) heard or interpreted was not the intended message.

Another important professional activity is helping two people who are continually interacting to shift from sarcastic to affirmative feedback. Under conditions of persisting criticism (e.g., when a father negates everything his daughter does), the daughter tends to stop listening and the communication cycle is disrupted in ways detrimental to both participants. On the other hand, supportive feedback is basic for the evolution of a trusting relationship with another human being or with the immediate environment (Erikson 1950).

Sometimes the worker can accomplish wonders by finding ways to unblock feedback which is, in fact, not able to return (Warfel, Maloney, and Blase, 1981). This is particularly true of shy or upset children who cannot communicate in spoken words but will do so in drawings or song. Similarly, when executives in a highly bureaucratic agency receive activity reports, the message has usually been "sweetened" by each level of subordinates on its way up, to the point that it no longer describes what is actually happening in the field. Such administrators, like political officials, can learn much by relying on a range of feedback channels. If they can be persuaded to listen to citizens as well as colleagues, subordinates, and the media, they may be able to avoid costly mistakes.

According to Vickery (1974) and Forder (1976), precise feedback is essential for enhancing the communication process. For example, in helping a youngster on probation, the social worker (the action system) will base her inputs on accurate feedback regarding

FIGURE 5.4. Feedback in Action

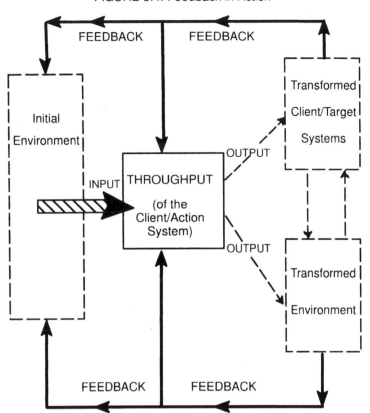

the youngster's throughput (resistance or internalization of advice) in the past, as well as on how court-derived outputs influence the target system (the probationer) over a period of time. In a rehabilitation process like that of the P. family, the client system (Mrs. P.) should become aware of the impact of this process on the primary target (i.e., herself), on other targets (e.g., her younger daughter), and on the environment (the public school from which the inputs about the daughter's failing grades originated). Other systems in the environment (e.g., the welfare office or the mental health clinic) might take steps to stay informed regarding changes in the P. family by participating in a case conference.

It can be quite a challenge for any social worker to manage a complex network of communication/feedback. Like the operator of a telephone exchange, the intervener must enable the entire system to function and serve as a link between units not yet functioning in a meaningful transmitter-feedback relationship. The same worker will have to perform a wide range of professional roles during any normal intervention effort.

INFLUENCING POLICY

In addition to becoming experienced with the methods of clinical practice, every social worker should feel equipped to apply the principles of systems analysis to making an impact at the policy level. Figure 5.5 depicts one way of launching into this topic. In a democracy, the population of any community consists of citizens who vote for candidates from the various political parties every few years and who, in the long run, become the elected official's constituency. Those elected to office engage in politics as a legitimate way to compete for authority and otherwise determine public norms for a designated period of time. The winner in politics is expected to use power and activate both centralized and decentralized public services judged to be the responsibility of government. Of course, these policymakers come to decisions under pressure from various interest groups, citizen organizations, agency professionals, regional planners, lobbyists, etc.

In a three-layer model similar to the political one, some community residents become the consumers of local social services, and many serve as laypersons or volunteers in the welfare field. Agency workers help grass roots, voluntary, public, and government representatives create more inclusive local participation. Participatory processes within welfare actually parallel the political ones that take place within government circles. Like others, social workers make efforts to influence agency policies as well as achieve implementation of specific policies through public services and voluntary bodies. Finally, local consumers of these services express satisfaction or impatience with the public services when they function as voters—and the circle is completed.

FIGURE 5.5. Social Work and Political Patterns of Influence

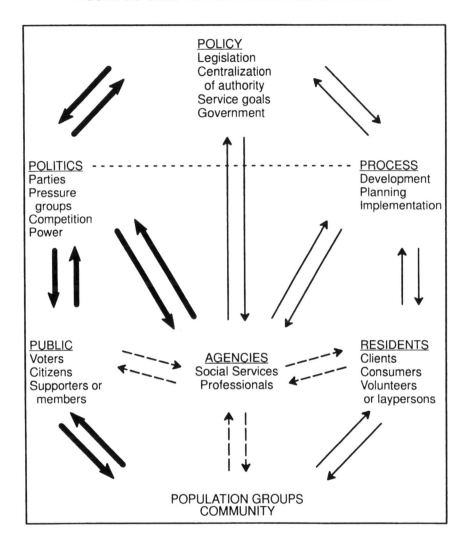

One way to utilize feedback cycles to influence policy is to strengthen the horizontal processes of a community system. For example, links could be forged between agency publics and the politician's constituents, or between practicing politicians and agency professionals. Even vertical channels can be enhanced if local branches are encouraged to communicate candid feedback to their own national office or to central offices of government. Local agencies would improve their functioning if they were to invite consumers (as well as local citizens who are not using their services) to give them feedback regarding what is actually happening out in the field. Of course, self-help groups and grass-roots organizations are based almost entirely on healthy horizontal interactions.

Figure 5.5 also indicates how agency personnel may try to influence policymakers in a reverse of the vertical pattern of accepting directives "from above." Two common activities in this vein are organizing citizen protest (marches with banners and blaring loudspeakers) against some undesirable situation, or lobbying for something which is strongly desired. Implementation efforts, such as social action or advocacy, involve a small, coherent group trying to change the functioning of a specific target within the constraints of a relatively short deadline. If the client system is willing to suffer a measure of public exposure, it may become involved in confrontation, conflict, or disruptive activities to promote a desired policy or oppose the enactment of an undesirable one in its environment (Miller 1988).

The following case history from Israel is illustrative.

Lobbying at the Legislature: A Case Report

During the spring of 1977, all of Israel's news media reported an increased incidence of rape. The police, under general criticism at the time, were seen to be handling rape cases poorly. Social workers became concerned when victimized women began asking for help at mental health clinics or appealing directly to well-known female members of parliament rather than reporting their experiences to the police.

Thus, at the beginning of July, the Executive Director of the Israel Association of Social Workers wrote to the Ministry of Interior (responsible for police services) suggesting that volunteer social workers be added to police teams sent to help rape victims. Within weeks, the Association and the police began the delicate process of learning to work together—and both received support for these efforts in the news media. A parliamentary subcommittee began hearings on revising all legislation dealing with rape problems.

The Association's Social Policy Committee prepared a set of recommendations by mid-December of the same year that stressed the social and emotional aspects of a proper crisis service for women who had been raped. These recommendations were well received by both police officials and legislators. Association representatives were invited to all meetings of the legislative subcommittee and were able to make an impact on the legislative changes which emerged (Kleinkauf 1981).

Within the next six months, the Association recruited volunteers from its senior members, trained them to work with police officers, provided supervision, collected reports, etc. Since there were no public expenses, the cooperation of all relevant government bodies was obtained. Volunteer social workers continued as part of this demonstration project until mid-1978, and their contribution was noted in many police as well as news media reports.

Once the revised legislation was passed, the Association made certain that key bureaucrats (in public and voluntary settings) implemented it, and that various population groups knew how to make use of the new services now available. After a two-year period, evaluative efforts confirmed that the counseling service was functioning well and was meeting the needs for which it had been designed.

Comments

The above story is from an Israeli reality, but attempts to do social action/lobbying/advocacy in other countries suggest many similarities. For example, the rather massive inputs required to bring about legislative change (outcomes) become clear when you look at the many tasks (throughputs) of the professional lobbyist (Brager 1968, Chetkow-Yanoov 1968, Gheluwe and Barber 1986). Although most of the work is time-consuming drudgery, successful lobbying is based on building trust relationships with all interested parties, supplying information to legislators, writing basic speeches for friendly politicians, and helping draft first versions of proposed laws as well as testifying at hearings. Lobbyists monitor (i.e., stay alert to feedback regarding) a bill's progress through the legislative process, helping it when possible or at least preventing interference by others. Sponsors are kept informed by means of a regular newsletter (feedback) as well as crisis-related telephone networks (Ashford, Macht, and Mylym 1987, Staut 1985).

In fact, when a bill reaches a crisis stage, lobbyists must be able to rally large-scale support from citizen and agency personnel populations. It is advisable to keep channels open to the opposition party (another version of feedback) and utilize every aspect of the legislative process with precision and sophistication (Dear and Patti 1981).

Of course, exerting pressure on policymakers must be done with the correct target system. For example, in order to raise the level of assistance for aged citizens, one must know whether to pressure service-giving organizations (agencies), policy or budget-allocating bodies (the Treasury or the United Way), and/or other influential persons or organizations (the Manufacturers' Association, the clergy, a planning body, organized consumer groups, etc.). Change agents who are responsible for lobbying must prepare intervention strategies appropriate to each target.

SUMMARY

In this chapter, you had the opportunity to test the applicability of systems concepts to a variety of micro and macro practice situations. You should now be comfortable with such ideas as client, target, and action systems; the five stages of any episode or project; and a range of professional roles. If you find merit in systems analysis, you should be able to describe deliberate change efforts in terms of managing inputs, boundaries, throughputs, and feedback.

In the next chapter, you can try to apply some of these systems ideas to understanding conflicts and to the efforts made to resolve them.

EXERCISES

Exercise 1: Defining a Problem

Please try to answer the following questions regarding one of your regular intervention efforts (e.g., with a multiproblem family, a faltering agency, an institutionalized older widow, the rapid spread of lice in schoolchildren's hair):

- As precisely as possible, what was the nature of the situation?
- What were the major causes of this problem or need situation?
- What change goals did you set for yourselves?
- What have you been doing about this situation?
- What was the outcome of your intervention?
- Would you judge that your efforts were successful?

Exercise 2: Distinguish the Apples from the Oranges

Suggest the appropriate client, action, and target systems for an episode of personal or family counseling as well as a session of the United Fund's allocation committee. Table 5.1 might help you to sort out your answers. Does focusing on target systems help you to sharpen your professional practice? If so, please explain.

TABLE 5.1. Client, Action, and Target Systems

	Marriage Counseling	**Allocating Funds**
Client System	_____	_____
Action System	_____	_____
Target System	_____	_____

Exercise 3: Describing an Episode from Your Workload

Based on a successful episode from your workload or from your involvements as a citizen, describe what happened in light of the following five action phases:

1. Initial environment
2. Creation of client system and specification of the target system

3. Expansion into an action system
4. Implementation
5. Transformation

Refocusing on the above episode, or on one of the case histories presented in this book, indicate how you might play one or more of the following professional roles:

1. Guide or stimulator
2. Consultant or expert
3. Enabler
4. Implementer

If your project did not require all the above roles, indicate which one(s) were missing and explain how this came about.

Exercise 4: Boundary Management in Your Workload

Drawing on problem situations with which you are familiar, illustrate the following two kinds of interventions: (1) opening up a closed boundary; (2) sealing a boundary more tightly.

What similarities or differences in professional activity did you find when trying to open a boundary to new inputs versus closing it to such an eventuality?

Exercise 5: Looking at Feedback in Your Workload

Taking another look at the Consultant's Report in Chapter 4, or at one of your own recent intervention efforts, suggest ways to make a deliberate impact on inputs, throughputs, and feedback.

Chapter 6

A Systems Model
of Conflict Resolution

INTRODUCTION

Conflict resolution is an important goal for all professional social workers. In fact, Lingas (1988) defined social work as "a harmony-building profession," claiming that client crises are often caused by unresolved conflicts and blocked communications. Other scholars have emphasized the importance of studying conflict professionally. For example, Chin (1961) analyzed the change process as the product of a system's efforts to achieve tension reduction. Burton (1984) claims that all conflicts begin in unmet human needs and unsatisfying human relationships. Similar sentiments are found in Purnell (1988).

It follows that many social work problems are rooted in intra- or intersystemic conflicts and that these might well be the outcome of changes in the system and/or its environment (see the input factors analyzed in Chapter 4). Whiteman, Fanshel, and Grundy (1987) analyze how to deal with angry parents, Warren and Hyman (1966) discuss consensus and dissensus in cases of community change, Weingarten (1986) advocates mediation for cases of marital conflict—and so on.

If you rely on a systems model of social work intervention, specific ways to resolve conflict need not be tied to any one method of practice. In fact, the following materials introduce a way of analyzing and dealing with conflicts which applies equally well in clinical, family, group, or community settings. This chapter suggests that a systemic model of four components is relevant for analyzing any persisting conflictual situation and for posing professional interventions appropriate for one component by itself or in combination with others.

SOME PRELIMINARY THOUGHTS ABOUT CONFLICT

Many scholars do not see conflict in negative terms (Coser 1956, Deutsch 1969, Warren 1969). New definitions of human nature, and analysis of conditions of affluence rather than scarcity, have produced a shift in conflict theory and a move toward the employment of systemic paradigms (Burton and Sandole 1986). In fact, a systems approach to analyzing conflict and conflict resolution implies:

1. Conflicts may be functional for a human system. In the story of the P. family (or of the recreation center), a certain level of tension, though creating a measure of discomfort, seemed essential for immediate survival. The existence of an active opposition is essential for preserving a political democracy. Thus, all conflicts should not be eliminated even if, indeed, that were possible. However, social workers would want to stop the escalation of conflict into destructive violence. They also want to focus on ways to de-escalate conflicts that have reached such levels.
2. The causes of most conflicts are multiple. Moreover, the causality operates in complex, circular (rather than linear) ways—as has been mentioned many times already. Consequently, a systems approach should be very helpful for understanding the many types of conflict we encounter in our personal and professional lives and for choosing our interventions appropriately.

FOUR COMPONENTS OF ALL CONFLICTS

Since all variables in a normal system interact continuously with all the system's other variables, it is difficult to think in conventional cause-effect terms. In fact, each variable can simultaneously be both a cause and a result. In the following material, we deliberately talk of components rather than causes. It is argued that all conflicts, from the smallest to the largest, include at least four essential components. These might be best understood as part of a comprehensive components-system-environment model. This possibly is elaborated upon in Figure 6.1 and in the text which follows.

FIGURE 6.1. The Four Components of Every Conflict

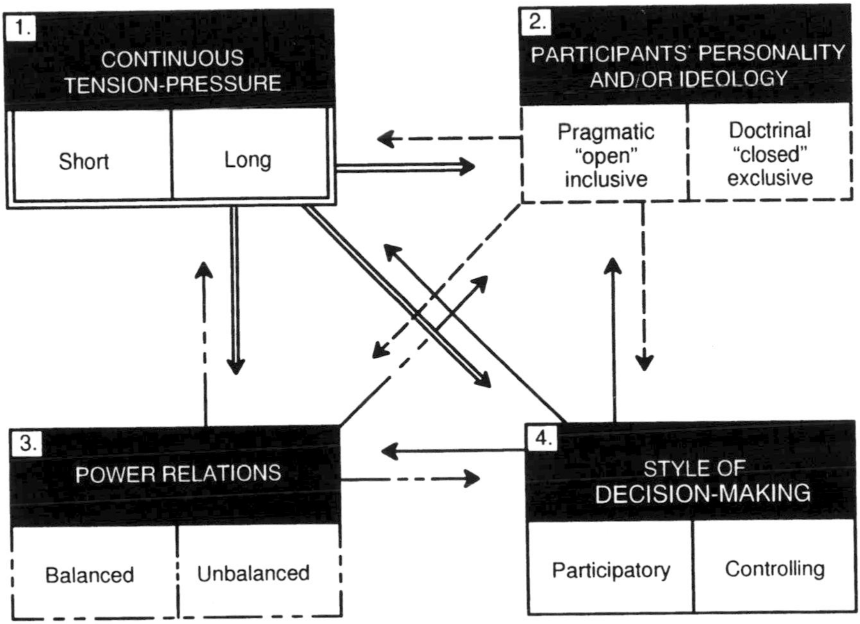

Continuous Tension/Pressure

Continuing conditions of pressure and/or tension in the environment penetrate through an increasingly permeable boundary to force a human system into a condition of input overload. As situational demands exceed the system's throughput capacity, outputs diminish and the mutual support function becomes numbed. The system's former steady-state interaction with its environment is disturbed, causing individual human beings or groups to feel stress or experience "crisis."

Such a crisis is usually of limited duration. In other words, people in crisis feel helpless or inadequate for, say, a few months, and then begin to recover (as they do after mourning the loss of a loved one). The problem is complicated when the crisis situation persists for a long period of time and causes either significant erosion of mental health or burnout. Exhausted persons cope poorly, making for more tension.

In situations of unceasing tension, people systems often defend themselves by simplifying the world into dichotomous camps (e.g., "we" versus "them"), or excuse their behavior with the certainty that "all the world is against us." They tend to abandon the middle ground in various continua. As they become more and more polarized, their system tends to become more closed and they rely on a domination style of decision making within the system. Without significant relief from the tension, they may indeed experience burnout, leave the community/environment, or escalate into violence.

Personality and/or Ideology of the Participants

Long-lasting conflict is often accompanied by a change from pragmatic, inclusive, humor-filled, decentralized, or open behavior to a devotion to purity of ideology/principles, exclusiveness, centralization, and great seriousness. Systemically, participants in an ongoing conflict often make their boundaries less and less permeable by favoring the purity-exclusiveness option.

In recent history, such closed behavior is exemplified by the action style of the Ayatollah Khomeini. Similarly, when the very conservative Barry Goldwater was a candidate for the presidency of the United States, he came up with the slogan "Better dead than Red." In closed persons or systems, alternatives disappear and even bystanders must choose "for me or against me." Generally, the situation worsens if the participants are also ignorant of the characteristics and the norms of the opposing group. Then, both sides fall victim to rumors, generalizations, and stereotypes, and they tend to function in a decidedly self-righteous style.

Such closed-minded participants, or tightly closed systems, tend to dominate decision making, see the world in neat dichotomies, and generally exclude others as unworthy of consideration. When they also have a large amount of power, they can both frustrate most efforts to resolve any conflict and rationalize the use of violence against a persistent opponent.

Distribution of Power and Influence

Scholars such as Lingas (1988) or Weingarten and Leas (1987) emphasize the centrality of power in situations of long-lasting conflict. The course of a conflict is certainly influenced by competition for power, influence, or resources (i.e., for control over a system's production-distribution-consumption). In addition, Purnell (1988) and Eisler (1987) stress the differences between those power arrangements that are symmetric (all rivals are of similar strength, power is shared) and those that are not (one side is very strong, the others weak).

In the days of the great empires, the strong ruled and the weak were conquered or exploited. Even today, a powerful elite can control things paternalistically or manipulate the social control mechanisms of its subordinates. However, having the power to win wars, or to dominate family arguments, is not enough to guarantee peace. The loser's acquiescence may be short-term and certainly does not create trusting relationships. If the strong party is too oppressive, members of the dominated side may become embittered—especially if they justify their existence on the basis of increasingly closed boundaries. When the victim of today turns into a fanatic victimizer, conflicts may continue or expand.

Styles of Problem Solving

There are three styles of dealing with conflict: denial, domination, or activating others as partners. Denial, as in the story of the white and black schools, is not recommended. On the contrary, conflicts, like problems, have to be acknowledged before they can be resolved.

Authoritarian use of power does achieve quick results, but it also generates resentment which contributes to conflict intensification (as it did among the staff in the recreation center). This stance is rooted in suspicion, fear, contempt, and secrecy—the usual conditions for attaining obedience. Oligarchic privilege often masks racist exploitation and bureaucratic manipulation. Attempts to dominate and struggles for control are often behind the rising intensity of conflict within a family, between victimized ethnic groups, and among organizations.

On the other hand, widening opportunities for rivals to participate in a system's throughput activities or enjoy its outputs (as in food-buying cooperatives, interdisciplinary committees, or multiparty coalitions) constitute a sound basis for conflict resolution (Chetkow-Yanoov 1986, Perlman 1976). The benefits of client involvement in agency decisions or self-help processes have been amply documented (for example, Katan 1981). The participatory style is usually accompanied by ideological openness, shared power arrangements, and a readiness to coexist with others in a pluralist/complex world (Fallon 1974).

FIVE POTENTIAL OUTCOMES

Figure 6.2 helps clarify what happens when you work simultaneously with two of the above components (open-/closed-mindedness and symmetric/asymmetric power arrangements).* At least five outcomes are possible:

Near Consensus

Open-mindedness and balanced power can create an atmosphere of consensus. Through cooperation and sharing between power equals, each participant or group is happy with the outcome, since each has attained something desirable (called a win/win outcome) it could not have achieved alone. The story of the evolution of a court-based domestic counseling service exemplifies this consensus process at the community level. Similarly, consensus is the ideal basis for a family decision (after full discussion) regarding what to do together during summer vacation. Of course, even in this atmosphere of general agreement, a participant can express mild opposition by asking for clarification, requesting additional discussion time, or suggesting another vote. If cooperation continues to produce results which

---

*With regard to the first variable, numerous exercises indicate that the other two conflict components, shortness of duration and a cooperative decision-making style, correlate strongly with open-mindedness. Similarly, long-duration of conflicts and coercive decision-making match up with closed-mindedness of the participants. It follows that the derivation of five types of conflict outcomes can be done adequately by means of a four-cell table using power symmetry/asymmetry and only one of the other three variables. For the purposes of this analysis, I chose to use the variable open/closed-mindedness.

FIGURE 6.2. The Five Types of Conflict

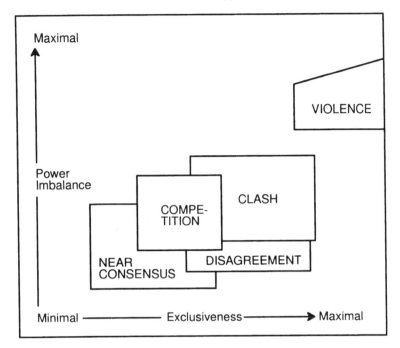

seem worthwhile to all the parties involved, cooperation will continue, and serious conflicts are unlikely to break out.

Competition

Open-mindedness together with power imbalance brings forth an atmosphere of competition. When the rules of the game require that one side lose, the stronger side will win, unless it decides to persuade all parties to agree with its desires by making an attractive offer (rather than risk losing in open competition). If the weaker side wants to win something and cannot invoke arbitration, it will have to strengthen its position or settle for less than it really wants. As in a tennis competition, the stronger player wins today, but in tomorrow's game, the former loser may rally and take back the prize. Adversary court procedures in which one party is judged guilty (or the fights in which Betty D became embroiled) take place in an atmosphere of competition.

Disagreement

Closed-mindedness and a balance of resources create an atmosphere of difference or dispute. In this situation, when highly principled players are not strong enough to dominate, they compromise. Most cooperation (as in political-party coalitions) "works" because the parties involved each lack sufficient power to operate independently (i.e., their participation in joint activities is understandably ambivalent).

Clash

In a situation of power monopoly and closed-mindedness, an atmosphere of dissensus can make for open clashes, as exemplified by the rivalry of the youth gangs in the poverty-stricken neighborhood of *West Side Story*. Such an atmosphere is equally typical of the Anglican decision to ordain female clergy, fights over ideological purity, protest rallies, and nonviolent rebellions. If the weak side is opposed in principle to compromise (as are fighters for freedom from colonial regimes), the price of keeping order escalates from year to year.

In an ongoing conflict of this type, if one side continues to lose, it may take on the characteristics of a victimized group. The distance between victimized groups and subsequent violence is small, and the episode is likely to move into the final option (described below).

Violence

In the event that the weaker side feels pushed to use violence and the stronger party engages in backlash (or counterviolence), both sides abandon accepted conflict norms and try to destroy the other. When election rivalries result in voters being killed, a protest rally degenerates into the looting of stores and shooting at the police, or the character of an opponent is assassinated in the news media, a conflict has escalated into violence. Under these conditions, the cost to both sides increases dramatically, and the likely outcome is one of lose-lose (Chetkow-Yanoov 1976 and 1987, Warren 1969, Weingarten 1986).

Closed minds/boundaries and an unequal distribution of power or resources seem to increase the risk of violence. The challenge is to devise intervention strategies which enable either a de-escalation from violence or the resolution of conflicts in their early stages, before escalation becomes serious. Thus, you may want to learn how to open up a closed system, or how to create a power balance by increasing a weak system's inputs of usable resources (discussed below). Again, you should find that the same principles are relevant to resolving conflicts among all types or levels of systems.

SELECTIVE INTERVENTION SUGGESTIONS

If you find the four components (described above) help you understand conflicts you have experienced, it should seem logical to examine types of professional intervention most appropriate for dealing with each of them. The following suggestions are based on my years of practicing conflict resolution in the United States and Israel as well as on the observations of such writers as Chandler (1985), Epstein (1970), Pearson and Thoennes (1985), and Warren (1964).

Dealing with Continuous Tension

In situations of ongoing tension, when a human system cannot close its boundary to tension-causing inputs or feedback from its environment, you first try to bring about some temporary relief. You might hold an unstructured discussion with tense people (where your ability to really listen is important) in order to ascertain their view of the situation, clarify their opinion about the components of this particular conflict, and provide an opportunity for catharsis. It is likely that they suffer from an accumulation of frustration, fear, and/or anger (some of the basic ingredients of burnout). Also, tense people may be trying to retain a modicum of psychological balance by denying that they are upset, or even that a conflict exists. Therefore, it is not advisable to start with interventions that might add to their sense of threat or burden. You might do better to begin with the problem as they see it and with empathy for their expression of feeling threatened, etc. Later, you can begin gentle questioning in order to help them face an uncomfortable reality.

Once a person or group can admit to having a problem which includes conflict, and that they are not coping well, you can initiate some problem-solving exercises. The latter might include the use of enjoyable techniques or experiences—in order to engender self-awareness, unrestricted thought, and skills learning (Chetkow-Yanoov 1987).

In addition to discussion, the emotional stress of conflict may be alleviated by such actions as:

1. using the large muscles (for example, in swimming or running) to achieve at least a temporary emotional relief by releasing some excess energy;
2. easing tension by means of drama, especially by the symbolic enactment of violence or tears on stage;
3. completing a mourning process, experiencing an act of forgiveness, or participating in a religious ceremony of reconciliation (These often help people achieve release from their former behavioral patterns as "slaves" or "victims.");
4. expanding mutual support by helping tense people laugh and relax in a supportive atmosphere of friends or neighbors; or
5. providing personal counseling if it is requested.

Confronting the Closed-Minded Person or Group

In some pluralistic democracies, laws are enforced against all closed-minded fanatics who disturb others in unacceptable ways. For example, you may have to start by disturbing a closed system's equilibrium by enacting new legislation (the social control function) against racism in order to make specific acts of bigotry or incitement punishable. Of course, coexistence behaviors (especially if they are new outputs for a formerly closed system) should be rewarded.

As above, while talking with a closed-minded person, listening carefully (even empathetically) is a prerequisite to initiating any meaningful change—in order to convince him/her that somebody cares. When the persons or groups involved have advanced beyond denial or fury regarding their condition, or when they have moved from righteous certainty to confusion or self-questioning, then giving them factual information (about the other side, etc.) may become appropriate.

You may be able to lessen, or prevent, the damage of a closed upbringing by either exposing all schoolchildren to basic instruction about a range of cultures and ethnic groups or by requiring them to learn at least two languages from nursery level (i.e., by opening up the system's boundaries to attractive vertical inputs). New intersystemic links, in the form of carefully structured educational encounters with members of other groups, are also useful (Rogers 1965).

Participation in a range of nonthreatening social activities can help create links between formerly segregated persons or groups. These could include joint:

1. participation in amateur musical, dance, or theater groups;
2. attendance at a performance which includes mixed-group discussions afterward;
3. participation in such groups for learning spoken English, handicrafts, carpentry, Japanese flower arranging, and the like;
4. volunteering together to help the elderly in their homes, those hospitalized in institutions, or those treated at emergency clinics; or
5. neighborhood improvement activities (in racially mixed environments) around the mutual desire to protect our schoolchildren from drug pushers.

Taking Action to Approximate a Balance of Power

In situations of power imbalance, the weak side may be strengthened by helping it increase knowledge, skills, assertiveness, access to funds, support and counseling, or access to the news media. The weak may also be defended by persons skilled in advocacy, by contacting the office of the public ombudsman, or by initiating an injunction in a local court of law (through the technology of social control). You might empower welfare clients by helping them organize for protest or for participation in a multigroup lobby favoring legislative change.

The very strong can be discouraged from abusing power by calling in the police, exposing their greed in a critical newspaper article, preserving an independent judicial system, or bringing a hidden controversy to public attention (in order to engender widespread discussion of the underlying issues). Such a sophisticated mixture of social control strategies can prove very effective.

Encouraging a Participatory Style of Problem Solving

If authoritarian decision making (i.e., a coercive style of using power to control other persons or systems) is detrimental to conflict resolution, what can be done to encourage a participatory style of interaction between rivals? You might invite leaders of competing groups or factions to a prestigious one-day, or a continuing, institute on methods of problem solving (Rouhana and Kelman 1994). By means of exercises and simulations (in a fun mode), these groups can experience how to solve problems without dominating and become familiar with such conflict-resolution strategies as forgiveness ceremonies, mediation, bargaining, and compromise—all in a supportive setting. By means of simulations and games, they might also experience both the costs of unrestrained competition and the satisfaction of finding answers to problems through joint effort. Suggestions for practical applications of these lessons in everyday life should be included.

The media could be encouraged to feature a series of leaders who are not authoritarian. It is also important that fictional heroes/heroines are seen to function successfully as enablers or peacemakers in a range of situational realities.

Participatory or collaborative strategies include being open to new ideas, providing information to all parties, enhancing open communications, stressing intergroup common interests, creating opportunities for horizontal interaction, engaging in necessary processes of mediation or bargaining, encouraging informal (vertical) contacts across boundaries, and demonstrating (to participants) that cooperation is worthwhile. The fact that such matters can be taught to grassroots citizens, schoolchildren, community leaders, professionals, and top administrators is demonstrated by the success of the Neighborhood Justice System in San Francisco (Chetkow-Yanoov 1976; 1986, Roderick 1987, 1988, Shonholz 1984).

Back in 1970, Epstein analyzed how role expectations seem to influence the orientation of social worker/change agents toward employing or avoiding conflict strategies. Professionals who are agency-oriented usually favor status quo norms and will avoid conflict. In contrast, an orientation toward clients has a radicalizing impact on professional norms, and such workers are comfortable using conflict strategies. Interestingly, orientation toward the profession is neither conservatizing nor radicalizing. Perhaps, with strong peer group support, profession-oriented workers might commit their expertise to the field of conflict resolution.

CONFLICT MEDIATION
AS A PROFESSIONAL ROLE

In Chapter 5, the "enabler" role was described in connection with one phase of an episode of system activity. The parallel role in conflict resolution is that of *mediator*. The mediator functions best in conflict situations where the disputants know each other, are accustomed to engaging in ongoing interactions, are still open-minded, and control similar amounts of power or resources. In such conditions, mediators try to reopen communications, enhance face-to-face contacts, help the rivals focus on specific issues, and (in an atmosphere of growing trust) encourage a free airing of differences. Gradually, distortions of "the facts" are lessened, and both sides realize that any settlement which they can agree to will have to be beneficial to both of them (Chandler 1985).

Like the *enabler*, a mediator tries to strengthen the healthy functioning of all participants until they are able—using a participatory process—to become responsible for solving the problem themselves. In contrast, *arbitrators* are authoritarian. They are most useful for conflicts in which the parties or systems have become closed and a power imbalance prevails.

The literature of mediation is so rich that a few examples should suffice here. Warren (1964) used his experience in mediating between East and West Germany to suggest that the mediator can be a change agent in most intersystem conflicts. Mediation has been used successfully to resolve disagreements between divorcing family members (Weingarten 1986), parties in child custody cases (Pearson and Thoennes 1985), neighborhood tensions (Shonholz 1984), and consumer-merchant disputes (Chandler 1985). Mediation was part of the role repertoire of the social worker who helped Mr. and Mrs. P. reduce their quarreling (in Chapter 2).

SUMMARY

In this chapter, you were asked to look at client problems as the outcome of unresolved conflicts. A systems model was introduced, focusing on four interacting components of any interpersonal, group, organizational, neighborhood, community-wide, national, or international conflict. Specific combinations of two components (systemic open- or closedness and symmetry or asymmetry of power) give rise to five types of conflict. Interventions for dealing with the various components (as well as types) of conflict were elaborated. The chapter closed with some observations on the social worker as mediator in conflict situations, tying this to an earlier analysis of the enabler role.

Now that you have used a systems paradigm to analyze people and environments, social change, practice issues, and conflict resolution, you might do well to look at how systems tools can help you focus on the professional practice of social work. Chapter 7 attempts to guide your efforts.

EXERCISES

Exercise 1: Checking on the Components of a Conflict

Describe a specific conflict in which you have been involved recently as a participant or intervener. How did any of the components (the conflict's duration, the participants' open- or closed-mindedness, the symmetric or asymmetric power realities, and authoritarian or participatory decision making) contribute to the conflict's evolution?

Did any of the above components act together, or show tendencies to act upon each other, in ways that caused the conflict to widen or undergo escalation?

Exercise 2: Resolving Conflict Through Tension Reduction

Does your personal or professional experience confirm that drawn-out conflicts tend to generate debilitating tension? Give an example from your workload, as follows:

- Describe the conflict.
- What were some of the negative consequences of the conflict?
- What did you do (can you do) to relieve the tension?
- How did/does tension reduction help resolve the conflict?

Exercise 3: Opening Up a Closed System

Does your personal or professional experience suggest that closed systems (which contribute to conflict intensification) can be helped to open up? Please suggest ways in which this was, or could be, accomplished within your caseload as follows:

- Describe the closed antagonist in your conflict.
- What did you do (can you do) to open the persons/system up?
- Did these interventions help resolve the conflict?

Exercise 4: Examining Other Conflict Resolution Interventions

In what ways does your professional experience suggest that bringing about a greater balance of power/resources or widening the opportunities for participation, or the two factors together, helps resolve conflicts?

- Describe the conflict situation.
- What did you do (can you do) to approximate a balance of resources?
- What did you do (can you do) to encourage participation?
- How did/do these interventions help resolve the conflict?

Exercise 5: Analyze a Conflict in History or in Literature

Please review the conflict between the two leading families of Padua (in the version by Shakespeare). If you were a consultant to the mayor of Padua, what would you advise him to do—so that the two families can stop feuding, and the story does not end with the tragic deaths of Romeo and Juliet?

Chapter 7

Implications and Conclusions

THE SYSTEMS MODEL AS PRACTICE THEORY

Throughout this book, you have been urged to adopt one specific systems model. Actually, this recommendation is part of an ongoing discussion in social work literature about espoused theory versus theory-in-use. Argyris and Schon (1974) present the issue well when they reason that successful people-helpers have a sense of what makes for competent practice, and that this is not deduced from basic theory but rather from reflecting and generalizing on successful clinical experiences.

All successful social workers are seen to build *their own* theory of practice on the basis of:

1. their accumulated experience with diverse problem situations or with specific human behaviors;
2. their memory of what, in past helping efforts, effectively brought about desired consequences;
3. their personal values and intuition; and
4. their selective adaptation of theories espoused by various scholars/colleagues.

Even though practice theory is seldom explicit, good practitioners tend to internalize abstract ideas and rely on them in meeting the action demands of everyday work.

According to Argyris and Schon, professionals will adopt a theory of practice if it meets some of the following criteria:

1. It makes client-worker interaction conducive to mutual learning.
2. Although it gives birth to recommended techniques, these remain open to improvement or correction as further experience accumulates.

3. It equips social workers for interacting with new kinds of clients/consumers as well as immersing themselves in a diversity of behavioral worlds.
4. It includes clues for reforming the profession, especially after a period of preoccupation with a specific ideology or practice technique.
5. It gives an intervener a sense of what real-world information is central (or peripheral) to specific helping situations.
6. It enhances the process (or artistry) by which a worker makes practice judgments in relation to dealing with those troubles for which clients request help.
7. It motivates clients to become more capable of accepting responsibility for their own lives.

These authors maintain that all professionals develop their own continuing theory of practice because it equips them to make diagnoses, design appropriate interventions, implement them, and test their effectiveness. Being grounded in sound practice theory is essential for guarding the profession against flaws and limitations that might cause it to suffer a crisis of legitimacy (Schon 1983).

The systems analysis model espoused in this book should, of course, be examined critically. It is recommended to you as compatible with the above criteria of sound practice and as enabling you to integrate practice ideas from many sources (Parsons 1988). The following review of the model's basic components should help you decide about making it part of your developing practice theory.

A REVIEW OF THE SYSTEMS MODEL

As a way to test how well you have grasped the systems approach, use some of the previous chapter's ideas on conflict resolution to analyze the following case history. A detailed checklist of system concepts is included at the end of the story, should you want to do a more thorough review.

Fighting the Establishment: A Case Report

In a small, urbanizing rural town, in a now ethnically mixed old neighborhood, one grade school's population totaled more than 1,000 pupils. The principal had been in charge of this school for twenty-eight years; in fact, most of the current teachers had once been his pupils. He was a tall, domineering person of considerable accomplishments, and a respected old-timer in the community. Although he gave lip service to the idea of parental involvement (by means of classroom and schoolwide committees), he was a one-man show. He had passed the legal age of retirement, but showed every intention of continuing in his post.

As the school year opened, several problems emerged. The chairperson of the school's PTO had not had any children in the school for three years. A heating problem in the school was tackled by the principal without consulting a parent who was a successful heating engineer, resulting in two weeks of darkness caused by an electrical fire. When the principal vetoed any parental involvement in setting up an afterschool recreation-study center, one activist parent became enraged. She had "had it with this small-time dictator" and vowed to take action.

She started by trying to communicate directly with the principal, but he remained indifferent to all her suggestions. When she finally organized an ad hoc committee of concerned PTO parents, and they initiated their own independent contacts with the town's education officials, the principal was furious. He opposed the activist at every private and public opportunity. He even sent her three threatening letters—first demanding conformity and later trying to buy her loyalty with promises. . . .

The activist and her group maintained that, in a democracy, no school principal may dictate to private citizens what to do; the group refused to disband or to be intimidated. Separately, each member continued to push for increased parental involvement in both administrative and, when appropriate, pedagogical school affairs. Most PTO meetings mirrored this clash of wills. During one end-of-the-year meeting, at which the principal behaved very patronizingly, the ad hoc neighborhood group walked out. Within days, a delegation of citizens gave the district superintendent of education a clear warning. If the principal did not retire immediately, the school would be paralyzed by a parents' strike next September, accompanied by a lot of negative publicity.

The message was understood and taken seriously. During the summer months, enough pressure was exerted on the principal to cause him to agree to retire at the end of the next year. The activist's group was satisfied, and the strike threat was withdrawn. Although the following school year was tense, the principal did leave at the end of the year, and he was allowed to retire with dignity.

Ironically, the activist, a much-sought-after speaker and consultant in human relations, was not invited to participate in any town activities for the next two years. It was as if she had been excommunicated.

Using three or four concepts from the discussion of conflict in Chapter 6, or from the concepts listed below, analyze the above case history in a systemic way. By now you should be able to do this with confidence.

Checklist of System Concepts

—System's boundaries
—Open or closed system
—Components of the system
—System's environment
—Horizontal relationships
—Vertical relationships
—Client system
—Action system
—Target system
—Feedback channels
—Linkage
—Steady state
—Inputs-throughputs-outputs
—Production-distribution-consumption
—Socialization
—Social control
—Mutual support
—Participation

—Systemic coherence
—Change agent

For example, you might analyze how the principal's closed-mindedness created social control outcomes that escalated the conflict; or, how the activist (the change agent) used feedback channels to limit the behavior of the principal (her target system).

MESHING EVERYTHING TOGETHER

In the first chapter, I hinted that one of the benefits of using systems analysis is that it makes possible for us to connect a wide diversity of factors or items into one complex whole—or to mesh everything together. Along with our appreciation of the power of intersystemic linkage, and that in reality many factors prove to be interdependent, perhaps we might be said to turn "meshianic." With such a paradigm in our heads and hearts, we can see the connection between radioactive waste, or the Chernobyl disaster, and the need to bury radioactively contaminated vegetables grown in the Middle East. We can also begin to speculate about the impact of some great leaders on many of the historic and cultural developments of their era. In this light, it seems very appropriate (these days) to note that we transmit and receive electronic mail on the world "net" or "web."

Figure 7.1 illustrates how systems analysis can help us understand a very complex reality by making a mesh of many relevant variables. If we remember the discussion of client and target systems in Chapter 5, this figure helps us see how their behaviors are intertwined differently in diverse types of conflict situations. When members of both the client system and its target systems are advised by a sophisticated change agent, they can learn which behaviors are appropriate in each type of conflict, and be able to avoid behaviors which will escalate the conflict into a more tense and costly variation. In fact, this figure may clue the change agent into suggesting specific behaviors which will lead to de-escalation.

In a somewhat different way, Figure 7.2 helps us make a mesh of grassroots, community, national, and international levels of agency functioning. Citizens, volunteers, and consumers of agency services

FIGURE 7.1. A Network of Client and Target System Behaviors in Four* Types of Normative Conflict

BALANCE OF POWER	IDEOLOGICAL POSITION	
	Open-Inclusive	**Closed-Exclusive**
Everyone Has Some (.5/.5)	CLIENT BEHAVIORS Communicate Participate Initiate Dialogue Consent Suggest Complain Cooperate Ask questions TARGET BEHAVIORS	CLIENT BEHAVIORS Compromise Cooperate Mediate Veto Bargain Appeal Boycott Accommodate TARGET BEHAVIORS
Strong vs. Weak (1/0)	CLIENT BEHAVIORS Convince Compete Debate Resist Sell Argue Arbitrate Convince TARGET BEHAVIORS	CLIENT BEHAVIORS Implement Subsidize Coerce Disrupt Punish Resist/Lobby Go to court Violate norms TARGET BEHAVIORS

*In a fifth opinion, both sides turn to violence (i.e., try to damage or destroy each other).

FIGURE 7.2. A Web of Vertical and Horizontal Interactions

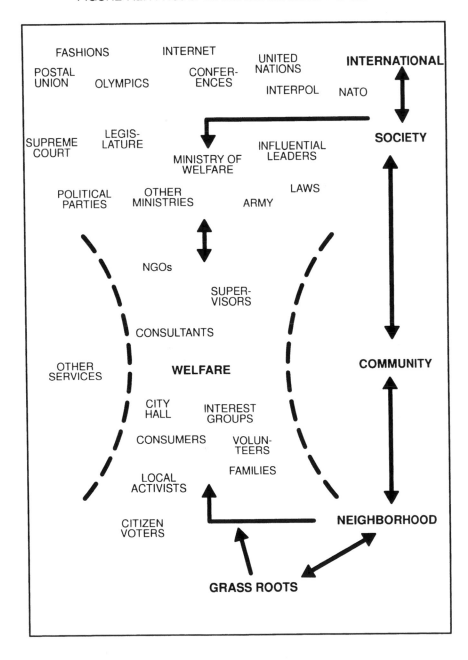

operate at the basic neighborhood level. They are tied into what goes on at the municipal Welfare office. It, in turn, has horizontal connections to other local agencies as well as vertical ones to its own national office. At that level, the head office is involved with other nationwide issues and actors. These, in their turn, have vertical international connections and horizontal ones with other national-level operations. In a democratic society, grassroots citizens become voters every few years. If they are happy with the services available, they will support municipal and national organizations, and these energies keep recycling. It is useful to see this phenomenon as a mesh or network.

LIMITATIONS OF SYSTEMS ANALYSIS

You are reminded that any system is a model, not a theory. Its concepts are derived inductively from how a part of reality works, and they may eventually help generate hypotheses for testing. However, you must be wary of enthusiasts who would have everyone believe that systems exist in some concrete form. A road map is never the road itself. You should, also, be cautious lest the tool which can shed light on our complex world be made into a faddish excuse for not thinking clearly (Mills 1959). In addition to these cautions, systems thinking should not be applied so rigidly (or so flexibly) that it loses all practical utility. Forder (1976) is particularly critical of social workers who liven up their talks or writings with a few references to systems, but who are simply playing with new jargon.

Rosenberg and Brody (1974) point to some of the difficulties of using a nearly value-free model like systems, especially within social and organizational settings that contain conflicting priorities. The model is said to miss part of reality due to its inability to predict the effect of actors' emotional involvements in any given situation. The very concepts and language of systems may, in fact, permit agency staff to disengage emotionally from difficult populations whom they are to serve. Neutral terminology, such as input overload or steady state, may actually allow practitioners to rationalize doing nothing about their agency's current program limitations.

Finally, Leighninger (1977) warns that making analogies should not be allowed to become another indoor sport. Any argument by analogy (e.g., the mind is like a switchboard, or coalition conflicts are like mathematical games) should be done with great care. He suggests that these aspects of the systems model be taken as hypotheses to be tested, but never as facts. He exaggerates, however, when he states that systems "may turn out to be another dead end for social work." By 1977, he should have known better.

USEFULNESS OF THE SYSTEMS APPROACH

As early as 1958, Hearn pointed out many ways in which systems analysis is relevant to the challenges that social workers face every day. He stressed the importance of understanding the individual-helper-environment network as a totality, focusing on prevention and crisis as well as on alleviation/rehabilitation. Aided by systems concepts, he found it very convenient to be able to conceive of individuals, groups, organizations, or communities as clients. He felt that social work should extend knowledge horizons, thus enriching its practice theory. Like engineers, consumers of assorted social science theories and research findings should be able to provide services that outlast the winds of fashion and the floods of overuse.

Systems thinking enables a flexible approach to understanding normal behavior and development by providing a functional versus dysfunctional axis for analyzing behavior. It helps practitioners grasp the entire helping network rather than remain partisan to one interventive method or preoccupied with clinically derived behavioral pathologies (Stein 1974).

Systems analysis can help practitioners understand and manage certain real-world dilemmas. For example, different types of action systems (e.g., caseworkers, nurses, remedial teachers, ombudsmen, or the police) can intervene with the same target system (e.g., a destructive gang of teenage boys). Conversely, the same action system might be appropriate for intervening with a number of target systems (e.g., individuals, families, groups, organizations, or neighborhoods) in one impoverished renewal area. When social problems are analyzed holistically, it is often possible to envision a full range of professional interventions—from prevention to restoration—with the same target system. Free from linear models of causality (formerly typical of the experimental sciences), practitioners can see behavior as a mosaic of interrelated components (Buckley 1968).

Interdependence and feedback are two central concepts in systems analysis. Some members of the helping professions are sophisticated users of positive reinforcement (i.e., feedback) in conditioning and socialization. Systems thinking emphasizes the contribution of every participant in the helping process to enabling or blocking the flow of vital information. It also clarifies that information and communicated knowledge are forms of power and can be utilized to cope effectively with economic or political forms of power (Chetkow-Yanoov 1968, Marcus 1979). Siporin (1975) indicates that systems analysis clarifies the multifunctional dimensions of "process" as well as stresses bridging or linkage concepts. He felt pleased to be released from the confines of method by such ideas as roles, tasks, functions, etc.

Pincus and Minahan observed that the systems approach is a conceptual framework that helps identify the professional tasks which must be accomplished after assessment and planning have been completed. Utilizing this model, you can grasp a number of regularly interacting variables and see them all as parts of a synergetic totality (Benedict 1970). In the long run, systems analysis supplies a frame of reference in which a unified model of social work intervention can be conceptualized.

Perhaps the core benefit of using the systems paradigm is that it has forced social workers to reexamine fundamental assumptions, extend knowledge horizons, and acquire new intervention skills. Siporin (1978) saw this as preventing the trained incapacity that takes place when a profession becomes overly institutionalized or subscribes so fully to one ideology that complacency sets in. Systems analysis constitutes an excellent example of what the social sciences can contribute to the enrichment of any practice profession.

ENVIRONMENTS
AND INDIVIDUAL DEVELOPMENT: CODA

Figure 7.3 summarizes many of the themes of this book. The central image is that the human being resembles a spinning top. As in systems analysis generally, reality is pictured as being in constant motion; in

FIGURE 7.3. Environmental Resources and Personal Development

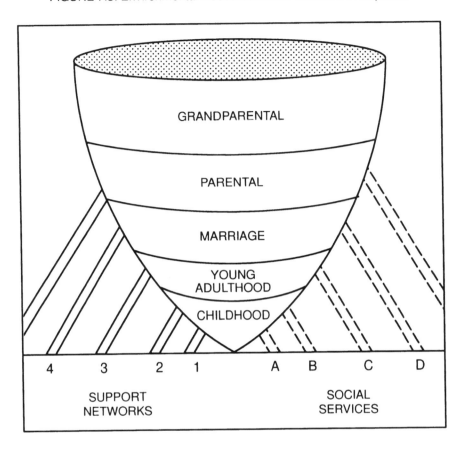

fact, motion helps living systems retain a dynamic stability while inactivity makes them fall into passivity and ineffectiveness.

A childhood rich with reciprocal relationships leads to growth and maturation. Artists such as Shakespeare, religious scholars, and social scientists have each postulated their models of ages and stages. They emphasize that there might be a certain order to human development and that each growth stage contributes to the successful completion of all other ones. When all stages have been enjoyed to the fullest, the "healthy top" will include many layers of complexity and will dance joyously for a full lifetime.

On the other hand, this active being may be a hollow shell. To counter such a possibility, two sets of environments are available to help the individual grow not only in size but also in maturity. The first, indicated by the numbers 1, 2, 3, 4, etc., at the left side of the top, are the natural helping or support networks discussed in earlier chapters. These include the following:

- Mother, father, siblings
- The total family
- Peer groups
- Neighbors and friends
- Work colleagues
- Acquaintances, colleagues, etc., from other countries.

They are all part of the growing individual's family and participant environments and operate through primary relationships to provide love, trust, nourishment, experiences, opportunities, challenges, responsibility, feedback about progress, etc. Blessed indeed is the youngster who grows up with all these supports intact.

However, many youngsters have to manage without a number of these natural supports. In the modern welfare state, formal social services provisions (letters A, B, C, D, etc., at the top right) substitute for the missing natural units. Operating on the basis of secondary relationships, society provides such private, voluntary, and public services such as:

- Mothers's helpers, homemakers
- Foster parents, adoption
- Public school classmates, youth club friends
- Neighborhood associations, block clubs
- Voluntary and public social service agencies
- Insurance, legislation

These arrangements become part of our community and national environments, often paralleling or replacing what should have operated in the natural network outlined above. Such social services as financial assistance, advice, lessons, enrichment, or medications— provided by an assortment of agencies—must become a part of any wholesome community.

FURTHER OBSERVATIONS
ON SYSTEMS-ORIENTED SOCIAL WORK

Asking social work practitioners and colleagues to base their professional practice on a systems analysis paradigm is not a simple matter. It does require effort to learn the concepts and language of systems analysis (the many exercises scattered throughout this book are intended to make this learning a little easier). Once the systemic way of thinking has become familiar, perhaps you will feel free to try it out in your practice.

Systems-oriented social work practice is based on the assumption that individuals or groups in need of service are not necessarily inadequate, deviant, or sick. Clients are defined as consumers whose service requirements fall within the normal behavior of all citizens. In fact, any person or group could become a client/target if they were the victims of prolonged input deprivation or feedback distortion. If the systemic imbalance or disruption that gave rise to their requiring help is remedied, they are presumed capable of acting in their own interests.

As in other models of practice, relationships are the foundation of successful living. A mother's loving behavior (her output) becomes the baby's input, just as the baby's feedback of contentment becomes the mother's new input. The complete message, like a fulfilling relationship, contains both objective content and affective connotations. If what was received is what the sender actually intended, trust relationships can flourish. Such experiences enable both sender and receiver to develop enough self-confidence to alter their own throughputs, take initiatives, accept added responsibilities, or help others. Together, all of these become the basis of a sound community (Gibb 1978).

Systems-based intervention also focuses on forging links among all relevant actors/systems; i.e., crossing boundaries that usually fragment the community. A professional worker will help a troubled consumer use a network of available services as well as gain access to each of them individually. As much as the workers are skilled in helping a dependent client, they should also be skilled in working with colleagues and superiors within the overall system-environment on the client's behalf. In an era of scarce and sometimes nonrenewable resources, the advantages of cooperative efforts (instead of exaggerated individualism and the fluctuations of market-oriented policies) should be high on every worker's list of priorities.

The systems model of practice remains attuned to commonly recognized social work ethics. The issue of confidentiality poses many difficulties, as the worker must decide to what extent information can be legitimately shared with other personnel who impact upon the target system's condition. As in most practice situations, the conflict between professional values and (employer) organizational allegiances must be faced. The matter is further complicated by the fact that systems-based practice involves the worker in many organizations. In order to engage in advocacy, many agonizing ethical decisions will have to be made—just as they would if utilizing any other model of social work practice.

Systems analysis can provide tools for moving toward an integrated micro-macro practice and helps specify the knowledge or skills required by the next generation of social workers. Systemic thinking offers another way to decide on the type of intervention to undertake. When you have become accustomed to seeing the problem in its totality, you will no longer be satisfied with partial answers. No systems-oriented professional will be satisfied, for example, with rehabilitating thirty drug users a year while another 500 addicts hit the streets during the same time period.

It is time to look at problems holistically, to offer assistance in a generalist manner, and to include prevention in everyone's daily repertoire. Systems thinking can help social workers reach such a goal.

Appendix A

The Systems Approach As a Model

INTRODUCTION

Anyone who has ever built a model boat or doll house knows how much beginners are helped when they begin with something that both approximates the larger reality and is also selective enough to be understood easily. Every model is not only a partial description of something, but also of how it works. If you observe children role-playing adventure stories, you are familiar with another type of modeling: that of testing out behaviors and their consequences in an interactive situation. Generally, what is learned from models and modeling helps you prepare for coping with the demands of life.

Scientists and professionals, like other human beings, use models in order to understand those situations in which they must take action or intervene. Such models are often created inductively, from accumulating experience. They constitute your image of what you want to study or to change (Loeb 1960). Professional practice, which takes place in the real world, involves actual people, behaviors, relationships, problems, and events (Beshers 1957, Meadows 1957). The systems model is one of the many tools available for understanding such behaviors and events.

PARADIGM SHIFT IN RECENT TIMES

Models of how the world is organized are often called paradigms. For example, until the Middle Ages, most people were convinced that the earth was flat and that the sun rotated around the earth. The story of its replacement by the paradigm of a round planet that rotated around the sun is well-known.

Certain paradigms have dominated human thinking over long periods of history. In our Western world, for example, a very powerful paradigm has been that used by the natural sciences and epitomized in the physics of Sir Isaac Newton. He and his peers thought the universe to be composed of inert matter (in a mechanical environment), space and time to be distinct, and causality to be sequential. As a result, phenomena could be studied experimentally by (supposedly) objective practitioners of the scientific method. A scientist was trained to analyze a problem, its component parts, and/or each part separately—a process usually called "reductionism." By the end of the nineteenth century, many academic disciplines (including biology, economics, and psychology) chose to be "scientific" in the manner of the natural sciences (Capra 1975, Checkland 1981, Forder 1976).

Since the 1950s, a new paradigm has become popular: that of systems. In contrast to earlier developments in the natural sciences, scholars began to view the world as a set of continuously interacting units and as a "whole" whose properties are much more than the sum of its component parts. Distinctions between space and time dissolve, as do those of matter and energy. Scholarly frameworks like nation/state are replaced by a postindustrial one of an ecologically interdependent planet. Natural resources cease to be viewed as inert matter, making for the evolution of models of abundance (and sharing) instead of earlier ones of economic scarcity (and hoarding). In fact, "information" is abundant and difficult to monopolize (Burton and Sandole 1986).

Instead of every problem having one clear cause (as when a specific germ/virus always causes the same illness), systems thinking recognizes that most human/societal conditions have multiple causes operating simultaneously. For example, a poverty-stricken neighborhood is seen as the outcome of such factors as illiteracy, crowding, weak family relationships, prolonged ethnic stigmatization of the residents, neglect by civic authorities, inadequate social services, etc. (not just because the poor "are" lazy and immoral). Not only do these many factors operate together to produce impoverishment, they also impact on each other as they interact. Actually, persons who use systems models understand that causes, interventions, and outcomes are in constant interaction. Yesterday's outcome might well be a causal factor in the dynamics of what is happening today.

THE BEGINNINGS OF SYSTEMS THINKING

Systems thinking has, of course, been around for many centuries. In theology, earth and the heavens were thought to be held together by such models as the wheel of fate or the music of the spheres. However, formal interest in systems analysis arose in the fields of physics and biology during the past sixty years (Woodger 1929, Cannon 1932, Von Bertalanffy 1940). By the 1940s, three important themes had penetrated the very core of systems analysis. First, an organismic metaphor of the universe replaced the former mechanistic one, shifting the emphasis from reductionism to a focus on living wholes. Second, the new science of information processing (cybernetics) enriched systems analysis with such concepts as input, output, and feedback (Stein 1974). Third, increasing attention was focused on open systems and their continuous interaction with their environments.

Checkland (1981) summarized the excitement generated by systems thinking in a model that shows how to conceive of an increasingly complex world. As he points out, any systemic level in his model contains all the properties exhibited by lower levels. As the level of complexity increases, it becomes difficult for an outsider to predict the system's behavior. His picture is seen in Table A.1. Checkland himself notes that humans, at Level 7, include all the properties of Levels 1-6, as well as the ones unique to Level 7 only. To put it humorously, if you kick a football (Level 2, a closed system), you pretty much know what will happen. The outcome is far less predictable if you kick a dog (a Level-6 open system). Incidentally, in the bottom right corner, where Checkland wrote "?" he might have inserted "mysticism" and "theology."

SYSTEMS THINKING IN THE SOCIAL SCIENCES

After World War II, systems thinking penetrated the social sciences through the works of such scholars as Lewin (1947),

TABLE A.1. A Continuum of System Levels

Level of Complexity	System Characteristics	Examples	Relevant Discipline
1. Structures, frameworks	Static	Crystals, bridges	Description only
2. Clockworks	Predetermined notion (may exhibit equilibrium)	Clocks, machines, the solar system	Physics, classic natural science
3. Control mechanism	Closed-loop control	Thermostats, homeostasis mechanisms in organisms	Control theory, cybernetics
4. Open systems	Structurally self-maintaining	Flames, biological cells	Metabolism, information theories
5. Lower organisms	Organized whole with functional parts, reproduction	Plants	Botany
6. Animals	A brain to guide total behavior	Birds and beasts	Zoology
7. Humans	Self-consciousness, knowledge	Human beings	Biology, psychology
8. Sociocultural systems	Roles, communication, transmitted values	Families, Boy Scouts, social clubs	History, sociology, anthropology, behavioral sciences
9. Trascendental systems	Unknowables	The idea of God	Theology, intuition, medication

Source: Adapted from Checkland (1981).

Homans (1950), Parsons (1951), and Loomis (1959). During the late 1950s and 1960s, systems analysis could be found in such diverse fields as sociology (Sanders 1958), medicine and psychoanalysis (Allport 1960, Menninger 1963), organizational analysis (Seiler 1967), education (Getzels 1960, Parsons 1959), engineering (Hall 1962), and planning (Kahn 1969, Moe 1960). The Society for the Advancement of General Systems Theory, founded in 1955, gave birth to numerous yearbooks and journals in subsequent years.

SYSTEMS THINKING IN SOCIAL WORK

Social work did not lag behind the above developments. Werner Lutz produced a summary of relevant social system concepts for the National Association of Social Workers of the United States in 1956. He borrowed ideas from other practice disciplines as well as the social sciences. Two years later, the systems-oriented approach of family therapists became popular among social caseworkers such as Ackerman (1958). In 1958, Gordon Hearn (who did his doctorate with Kurt Lewin at M.I.T. ten years earlier) wrote that "system" was a central construct or model for social work theorizing.

Also, in 1958, the systems content of Lippitt, Watson, and Westley's book *The Dynamics of Planned Change* rocked the therapy-oriented social work profession. These authors dared to analyze personality, groups, organizations, and communities with the same analytic tool: i.e., as systems. The concepts of power, communication, client system, and change agent became part of the professional vocabulary.

By 1961, William Schwartz was thinking about social groups as systems, Bennis and his colleagues were analyzing planned change in systems terms, and Sidney Zimbalist wrote about the problem of community equilibrium. Two years later, Roland Warren devoted a number of chapters of *The Community in America* (1963) to systems analysis, joining Lippitt as one of the seminal contributors to the development of community social work theory.

In 1968, Germain made one of the first attempts to apply some systems concepts in casework practice. One year later, Gordon Hearn's groundbreaking book *The General Systems Approach* was published. Among its many gems, the book included Shulman's look at system ideas in field instruction. In the same year, Janchill published an article on systems concepts in casework practice.

During the 1970s, social work publications based on systems analysis continued to multiply. Relevant contributions are found in such topic areas as social theory (Compton and Galway 1975), social group work (Klein 1972), service networks (Rosenberg and

Brody 1974), social planning (Goldberg and Neil 1972), social casework (Hartman 1970), and social policy (Hoos 1972).

In 1973, Kahn devoted part of a chapter to discussing what the systems framework might be able to contribute to shaping a new social work. During the same year, Goldstein as well as Pincus and Minahan published books on social work practice that rely extensively on systems concepts. Pincus and Minahan stressed that clients actually interact within complex networks of resource systems and social situations. They also widened the definition of intervention, indicating that every practitioner should be viewed as a change agent operating with client, target, and action subsystems. After reviewing the evolution of practice theory in social work, Goldstein stressed that the social worker and people in treatment actually constitute a single network or change system, and that their interactions include social preconditions as well as environmental contexts. Within the change system, the worker's primary effort is to facilitate exchange, communication, and learning at each stage of the problem-solving partnership.

Hearn wrote a chapter on "general systems theory and social work" in Turner's book *Social Work Treatment* (1974), and again in its 1979 revision. Siporin continued the approach in 1975 and 1978. Basing himself in ecological theory, he saw practice as based on eight systemic levels rather than still being categorized by methods. He recognized the systems underpinnings of human growth models like that of Erikson, and indicated an emerging paradigm shift within the profession—from clinical practice theories to a unified conception of social work practice based in the ecology model.

The list goes on and on.

Appendix B

Outline of a Suggested
One-Semester MA Course
on "Systems Analysis in Social Work"

LESSON NUMBER	BASIC LESSON	WHERE IN THE BOOK
1.	Models, paradigms, systems	Appendix A
2.	Definitions and concepts	Chapters 2-3
3.	Case histories:	
	The P. Family	Chapter 2
	Betty D.	Chapter 3
4.	Systems and environments	Chapter 1
5.	Conflict resolution theory	Chapter 6
6.	Conflict resolution applications	Chapter 6
7.	Systems and change	Chapter 4
8.	Recreation center case history	Chapter 4
9.	Client/action/target systems	Chapter 5
10.	Episodes of system activity	Chapter 5
11.	Managing inputs/throughputs	Chapter 3
		Chapter 5
12.	Feedback management	Chapter 2
		Chapter 3
		Chapter 5
13.	Social action:	
	Lobbying the legislature	Chapter 5
	Changing a public school	Chapter 7
14.	Summary and implications	Chapter 7

Bibliography

Ackerman, N. W., The homeostasis of behavior, *The Psychodynamics of Family Life*, New York: Basic Books, 1958, 68-79.

Ackoff, R. L., *Redesigning the Future: A Systems Approach in Societal Problems*, New York: Wiley, 1974.

Allport, G. W., The open system in personality theory, *Journal of Abnormal and Social Psychology*, 61(3), 1960, 301-310.

Anderson, R. E., and Carter, I. E., *Human Behavior in the Social Environment: A Social Systems Approach*, Chicago: Aldine, 1974.

Anner, S., *Report of the Consequences of the Economic Crisis for the Present and Future Development of Social Welfare*, Vienna: European Center for Social Welfare Training and Research, 1982, Eurosocial Report No. 17.

Ansbacher, H. L., A humanist consensus, *Journal of Humanist Psychology*, 18, Summer 1978, 87-92.

Argyris, C., and Schon, D. A., *Theory in Practice: Increasing Professional Effectiveness*, San Francisco: Jossey-Bass, 1974.

Ashford, J. B., Macht, M. W., and Mylym, M., Advocacy by social workers in the public defender's office, *Social Work*, 32, May-June 1987, 199-204.

Baker, F., Broskowski, A., and Brandwein, R., System dilemmas of a community health and welfare council, *Social Service Review*, 47, March 1973, 63-80.

Baker, R., Toward generic social work practice, *British Journal of Social Work*, 5, Summer 1975, 193-215.

Bebout, J. E., and Bredmeier, H. C., American cities as social systems, *Journal of the American Institute of Planners*, 29, May 1963, 64-76.

Benedict, R., Synergy: Patterns of the good culture, *Psychology Today*, 4, June 1970, 51-55, 75-77.

Bennett, J. W., *The Ecological Transition*, New York: Pergamon, 1976.

Beshers, J. M., Models and theory construction, *American Sociological Review*, 22, February 1957, 32-38.

Bloedorn, J. C., MacLatchie, E. B., Friedlander, W., and Wedemeyer, J. M., Designing social service systems, *Tactics and Techniques of Community Practice*, Eds. F. M. Cox, J. L. Erlich, J. Rothman, and J. E. Trapman, Itasca, IL: Peacock, 1977, 81-104.

Boulding, K. E., General systems theory—a skeleton of science, *Management Science*, 2, April 1956, 197-208.

Brager, G. A., Advocacy and political behavior, *Social Work*, 13, April 1968, 5-15.

Bronfenbrenner, U., *The Ecology of Human Development*, Cambridge, MA: Harvard University Press, 1979.

Brown, J. H., Finch, W. A., Northern, H., Taylor, S. H., and Weil, M. *Child, Family, Neighborhood: A Master Plan for Social Service Delivery*, New York: Child Welfare League of America, 1982.

Buckley, W., Ed., *Modern Systems Research for the Behavioral Scientist*, Chicago: Aldine, 1968.

Burton, J. W., *Global Conflict: The (Local) Sources of International Crisis*, Brighton (England): Wheatsheaf Books, 1984.

————. and Sandole, D. J. D., Generic theory: The basis of conflict resolution, *Negotiation Journal*, 2, October 1986, 333-344.

Calhoun, J. B., The role of space in animal sociology, *Journal of Social Issues*, 22, October 1966, 46-58.

Cannon, W. B., *Wisdom of the Body*, New York: Norton, 1932.

Capelle, R. G., *Changing Human Systems*, Toronto: International Human Systems Institute, 1979.

Capra, F., *The Tao of Physics*, Suffolk: Richard Clay, 1975.

Chandler, S. M. Mediation: Conjoint problem solving, *Social Work*, 30, July/August 1985, 346-349.

Checkland, P. *Systems Thinking, Systems Practice*, New York: Wiley, 1981.

Chetkow, B. H., Sectarian social work and the changing functions of formal religion, *Journal of Jewish Communal Service*, 39, Summer 1963, 358-367.

————. Some factors influencing the utilization and impact of priority recommendations in community planning, *Social Service Review*, 41, September 1967, 271-282.

_____. The planning of social service changes, *Public Administration Review*, 24, May/June 1968a, 256-263.

_____. So go fight city hall, *Neighborhood Organization for Community Action*, Ed. J. B. Turner, New York: National Association of Social Workers, 1968b, 194-203.

_____. Conflict as the dynamics of power in the local community, *Social Work Today*, 7, July 1976, 238-240.

_____. Some notes on systems analysis of social work practice, *Contemporary Social Work Education*, 3, August 1980, 179-190.

_____. Short-term community intervention, *Stress and Anxiety*, Ed. N. A. Milgram, New York: Hemisphere Publishing Co. (McGraw-Hill International), Vol. 8, 1982, 287-301.

_____. Participation as a means to community cooperation, *Community and Cooperatives in Participatory Development*, Eds. Y. Levi and H. Litwin, Aldershot (England): Gower, 1986, 21-35.

_____. *Dealing with Conflict and Extremism*, Jerusalem: Israel Joint Distribution Committee, 1987.

_____. Conflict resolution skills can be taught, *Peabody Journal of Education*, 71(3), 1996, 12-28.

_____. *Social Work Approaches to Conflict Resolution*, Binghamton, NY: The Haworth Press, 1997.

Chin, R., The utility of system models and developmental models for practitioners, *The Planning of Change*, Eds. W. G. Bennis, R. O. Benne, and R. Chin, New York: Holt, Rinehart & Winston, 1961, 201-214.

Cho, S. A., Freeman, E. M., and Patterson, S. L. Adolescents' experience with death: Practice implications, *Social Casework*, 63, February 1982, 88-94.

Compher, J. V., Parent-school-child systems: Triadic assessment and intervention, *Social Casework*, 63, September 1982, 415-423.

Compton, B. R., and Galway, B., General systems theory as a conceptual framework, *Social Work Process*, Homewood: Dorsey Press, 1975, 60-73.

Coser, L. A., *The Functions of Social Conflict*, Glencoe: Free Press, 1956.

Coulton, C. J., Person-environment fit as the focus in health care, *Social Work*, 26, January 1981, 26-35.

De Hoyos, G., and Jensen, C., The systems approach in American social work, *Social Casework*, 66, October 1985, 490-497.

Dear, R. B., and Patti, R. J., Legislative advocacy: Eleven effective steps, *Social Work*, 26, July 1981, 289-296.

Deutsch, M., Conflicts: Productive and destructive, *Journal of Social Issues*, 25, January 1969, 7-41.

Doig, J. W., Police problems, proposals, and strategies for change, *Public Administration Review*, 28, September/October 1968, 393-406.

Drabeck, T. E., and Haas, J., Laboratory simulation of organizational stress, *American Sociological Review*, 34, April 1969, 223-238.

Duhl, L., Planning and predicting: Or what to do when you don't know the names of the variables, *General Systems Theory and Psychiatry*, Eds. W. Gray, J. W. Fidler, and J. R. Bottísta. Boston: Little, Brown, 1969, 337-346.

Ehrlich, G., In New Mexico: (Alan Savoy) Desert Healer, *Time*, December 7, 1987.

Eisenhart, R. W., Flower of the dragon: An example of applied humanistic psychology, *Journal of Humanistic Psychology*, 17, Winter 1977, 3-24.

Eisler, R., The essential difference: Crete and memories of a lost age, *The Chalice and the Blade*, San Francisco: Harper & Row, 1987, 29-41 and 133-155.

Elgin, D., *Voluntary Simplicity*, New York: Bantam Books, 1982.

Emery, F. E., and Trist, E. L., The causal texture of organizational environments, *Human Relations*, 18, 1965, 21-31.

Engel, G. L., The clinical application of the biopsychosocial model, *American Journal of Psychiatry*, 137, May 1980, 535-544.

Epstein, I., Professional role orientations and conflict strategies, *Social Work*, 15, October 1970, 87-92.

Erikson, E. H., Eight stages of man, *Childhood and Society*, New York: Norton, 1950, 219-234.

Fallon, K. P., Participatory management, *Child Welfare*, 53, November 1974, 555-562.

Fischer, J., The social work (knowledge) revolution, *Social Work*, 26, May 1981, 199-207.

Forder, A., Social work and systems theory, *British Journal of Social Work*, 6, Spring 1976, 23-42.

_____. The systems approach and social work methods, *Social Work Education*, 1, Spring 1982, 4-10.

Fraley, Y. L., A role model for practice, *Social Service Review*, 43, June 1969, 145-154.

Freed, A. O., Building theory for family practice, *Social Casework*, 63, October 1982, 472-481.

Fromm, E., *Escape from Freedom*, New York: Holt, Rinehart & Winston, 1941.

Fuller, R. B., *Synergetics: Explorations in the Geometry of Thinking*, New York: Collier Books of Macmillan, 1975.

Fuller, T. K., Social factors and mental hospitalization, *Social Work*, 22, March 1977, 151-153.

Germain, C. B., Social study: Past and future, *Social Casework*, 49, July 1968, 403-409.

_____. An ecological perspective in casework practice, *Social Casework*, 54, June 1973, 323-330.

_____. General systems theory and ego psychology, *Social Service Review*, 52, December 1978, 535-550.

_____. Human development in contemporary environments, *Social Service Review*, 61, December 1987, 565-580.

_____. The place of community work within an ecological approach to social work practice, *Theory and Practice of Community Social Work*, Eds. S. H. Taylor and R. W. Roberts, New York: Columbia University Press, 1985, 30-55.

Getzels, J. W., and Thelen, H. A., The classroom group as a unique social system, *The Dynamics of Instructional Groups*, Ed. N. B. Henry, Chicago: University of Chicago Press, 1960, Vol. 2, 65-82.

Gheluwe, B., and Barber, J. K., Legislative advocacy in action, *Social Work*, 31, September/October 1986, 393-395.

Gibb, J. R., *Trust: A New View of Personal and Organizational Development*, Los Angeles: Guild of Tutors Press, 1978.

Gilmore, T. N., Leadership and boundary management, *Journal of Applied Behavioral Science*, 18(3), 1982, 343-356.

Goldberg, E. M., and Neil, J. E., Collaborating with other agencies, *Social Work in General Practice*, London: Allen & Unwin, 1972, 146-162.

Goldstein, H., *Social Work Practice*, Columbus: University of South Carolina Press, 1973.

Gordon, W. E., A natural classification system for social work literature and knowledge, *Social Work*, 26 March 1981, 134-138.

Gotteschalk, S. S., A definition of community, *Communities and Alternatives*, London: Wiley, 1975, 18-24.

Gouldner, A. W., Anti-Minotaur: The myth of a value-free sociology, *Social Problems*, 9, 1962, 191-213.

Green, R. G., A survey of family therapy practitioners, *Social Casework*, 63, February 1982, 95-99.

Greenwood, E., The practice of science and the science of practice, *The Planning of Change*, Eds. W. C. Bennis, K. D. Benne, and R. Chin. New York: Holt, Rinehart & Winston, 1961, 73-82.

Greer, S., Normative theory and empirical theory, *The Logic of Social Enquiry*, Chicago: Aldine, 1969, 177-185.

Hall, A. D., *A Methodology for Systems Engineering*, Princeton: Van Nostrand, 1962.

Hall, E. T., *Distances in man, The Hidden Dimension*, Garden City: Doubleday, 1966, 107-122.

Hartman, A. To think about the unthinkable, *Social Casework*, 51, October 1970, 467-474.

————. Diagrammatic assessment of family relationships, *Social Casework*, 59, October 1978, 465-476.

————. An ecologically oriented systems approach to helping families, *Working with Adoptive Families Beyond Placement*, New York: Child Welfare League of America, 1984, 11-21.

————. *Practice in adoption, A Handbook of Child Welfare*, Eds. J. Laird and A. Hartman, New York: Free Press, 1985, 667-692.

Hashimi, J. K., Environmental modification, *Social Work*, 26, July 1981, 323-326.

Hawley, A. H., *Urban Society: An Ecological Approach*, New York: Ronald Press, 1971.

————. *Societal Growth: Processes and Implications*, New York: Free Press, 1979.

Hearn, G., *Systems: The central construct, Theory Building in Social Work*, Toronto: University of Toronto Press, 1958, 38-51.

————. Ed. *The General Systems Approach*, New York: Council of Social Work Education, 1969.

_____. Social work as boundary work, *Iowa Journal of Social Work*, 3(2), 1970, 60-64.

_____. General systems theory and social work, *Social Work Treatment: Interlocking Theoretical Approaches* (1974), Ed. J. Turner, New York: Free Press, 1979, 333-359.

Heath, A., *Rational Choice and Social Exchange: A Critique of Exchange Theory*, New York: Cambridge University Press, 1976.

Henderson, H., Living earth's lessons, *One Earth*, 8, Spring 1988, 4-5 and 30-32.

Holmberg, A. R., Participant intervention in the field, *Human Organization*, 14, Spring, 1955, 23-26.

Homans, G. C., The external system, and the internal system, *The Human Group*, New York: Harcourt Brace, 1950, 108-155.

Hoos, I., *Systems Analysis in Public Policy*, Berkeley: University of California Press, 1972.

Jackson, D. D., The question of family homeostasis, *Psychiatric Quarterly Supplement*, 31, 1957, 79-90.

Janchill, M. P., Systems concepts in casework theory and practice, *Social Casework*, 50, February 1969, 74-82.

Jantsch, E., Ed., *The Evolutionary Vision: Towards a Uniting Paradigm of Physical, Biological, and Sociocultural Evolution*, Boulder, CO: Westview Press, 1981.

Kahn, A. J., *Theory and Practice of Social Planning*, Beverly Hills: Sage, 1969.

_____. A systems framework, *Shaping the New Social Work*, New York: Columbia University Press, 1973, 47-52.

Kasarda, J. D., The structural implication of social system size, *American Sociological Review*, 39, February 1974, 19-28.

Katan, Y., Patterns of client participation in local human service organizations, *Social Development Issues*, 5, Summer/Fall 1981, 134-150.

Katz, D., and Kahn R., *Systems Thinking*, Ed. F. E. Emery, Middlesex: Penguin Books, 1969.

Katz, E., Lewin, M. L., and Hamilton, H. Traditions of research on the diffusion of innovation, *American Sociological Review*, 28, April 1963, 237-252.

Kepner, E., Gestalt group process, *Beyond the Hot Seat: Gestalt Approaches to the Group*, Eds. B. Federer and R. Ronall, New York: Brunner/Mazel, 1980, 5-23.

Kirk, S. A., Clients as outsiders: Theoretical approaches to deviance, *Social Work*, 17, March 1972, 24-32.

Klein, A. F., A group as a social system, *Effective Groupwork*, New York: Association Press, 1972, 125-133.

Kleinkauf, C., Guide to giving legislative testimony, *Social Work*, 26, July 1981, 279-303.

Kluckhohn, C., *Navaho Witchcraft*, Cambridge: Peabody Museum, Paper No. 22, Vol. 2, 1944.

Kuhn, A., and Beam, R. D., *The Logic of Organization: A System-Based Social Science Framework for Organization Theory*, San Francisco: Jossey-Bass, 1982.

Lauffer, A., *Assessment Tools for Practitioners, Managers, and Trainers*, Beverly Hills: Sage, 1982.

Laves, R. G., Contact and boundary: Creating a nontraditional college classroom, *Beyond the Hot Seat: Gestalt Approaches to Group*, Eds. B. Federer and R. Ronall, New York: Brunner/Mazel, 1980, 155-166.

Leighninger, R. D., Systems theory in social work: A reexamination, *Journal of Education for Social Work*, 13, Fall 1977, 44-49.

Lewin, K., Field theory and experiments in social psychology, *American Journal of Sociology*, 44, May, 1939, 868-896.

———.Quasi-stationary social equilibria and the problem of permanent change, *The Planning of Change*, Eds. W. G. Bennis and Others, New York: Holt, Rinehart & Winston, 1961, 235-238.

———. Feedback problems of social diagnosis and action (1947), *Modern Systems Research for the Behavioral Scientist*, Ed. W. F. Buckley, Chicago: Aldine, 1968, 441-445.

Lieber, A. L., *The Lunar Effect: Biological Tides and Human Emotions*, New York: Anchor/Doubleday, 1978.

Lingas, G. L., Conflict resolution within family and community networks, *Nordic Journal of Social Work*, 8, 1988, 48-58.

Lippitt, R. L., Watson, J., and Westley, B. *The Dynamics of Planned Change*, New York: Harcourt & Brace, 1958.

Loeb, M. B., The backdrop for social research: Theory-making and model building, *Social Science Theory and Social Work Research*,

Ed. L. S. Kogan, New York: National Association of Social Workers, 1960, 3-15.

Loomis, C. P., Systemic linkage in El Cerrito, *Rural Sociology*, 24, March 1959a, 54-57.

————. Tentative types of directed social change involving systemic linkage, *Rural Sociology*, 24, December 1959b, 383-390.

————. and Beegle, J. A., Social systems and social change, and Locality systems, *A Strategy for Rural Change*, New York: Schenkman, 1975, 1-60.

Lutz, W. A., *Concepts and Principles Underlying Social Work Practice*, New York: National Association of Social Workers, 1956.

Marcus, L., Communications concepts and principles, *Social Work Treatment*, Ed. F. J. Turner, New York: Free Press, 1979, 409-432.

Masow, A., The role of basic need gratification in psychological theory, *Motivation and Personality*, New York: Harper & Row, 1954, 80-106.

Meadows, P., Models, systems, and science, *American Sociological Review*, 22, February 1957, 3-9.

Menninger, K., *The Vital Balance*, New York: Viking, 1963.

Merton, R. K., Manifest and latent functions, *Social Theory and Social Structure*, Glencoe: Free Press, 1957, 60-84.

Miller, G. T., Politics and environment, *Living in the environment* (1975), Belmont, CA: Wadsworth, 1988, 572-589.

Miller, J. G., Toward a general theory for the behavioral sciences, *American Psychologist*, 10, 1955, 513-531.

————. *Living Systems*, New York, McGraw-Hill, 1978.

Mills, C. W., Grand theory, *The Sociological Imagination*, New York: Oxford University Press, 1959, 25-49.

Mishne, J. M., The missing system in social work's application of systems theory, *Social Casework*, 63, November 1982, 547-553.

Moe, E. O., Consulting with a community system, *Journal of Social Issues*, 15(2), 1960, 29-35.

Moos, R. H., *The Human Context*, New York: Wiley, 1976.

Mott, B. J. F., *Anatomy of a Coordinating Council*, University of Pittsburgh Press, 1968.

Nowotny, H., *The Information Society*, Vienna: European Center for Social Welfare Training and Research, 1981, Eurosocial Paper No. 9.

Olsen, M., *The Process of Social Organization*, New York: Holt, Rinehart & Winston, 1968.

Ophuls, W., *Ecology and the Politics of Scarcity*, San Francisco: W. H. Freeman, 1977.

Parsons, R. J., Integrative practice: A framework for problem solving, *Social Work*, 33, September/October 1988, 417-421.

Parsons, T., *The Social System*, New York: Free Press, 1951.

———. The school class as a social system, *Harvard Education Review*, 29, Fall 1959, 297-318.

———. On building social system theory: A personal history, *Daedalus*, 99, Fall 1970, 826-881.

Pearson, J., and Thoennes, N., Mediation versus the courts in child custody cases, *Negotiation Journal*, 1, July 1985, 235-244.

Perlman, J. E., Grassrooting the system, *Social Policy*, 7, September/October 1976, 4-20.

Pincus, A., and Minahan, A., Four basic systems in social work practice, *Social Work Practice: Model and Method*. Itasca: Peacock, 1973, 53-68.

Portmann, A., Beyond Darwinism, *Commentary*, 40, November 1965, 31-41.

Prigogine, I., and Stengers, I., *Order Out of Chaos*, New York: Bantam Books, 1984.

Purnell, D., Creative conflict, *WCCI Forum*, 2, June 1988, 30-52.

Ramsay, R. F., Social work's search for a common conceptual framework, *Proceedings*, Tokyo, 23rd International Congress of Schools of Social Work, 1987, 50-56.

———. *Is Social Work a Profession?*, University of Calgary, July 1988, Mimeographed.

Reid, W. J., Problem formation and resolution, *The Task-Centered System*, New York: Columbia University Press, 1978, 42-82.

———. Mapping the knowledge base of social work, *Social Work*, 26, March 1981, 124-132.

Richmond, M. E., *What is Social Casework?: An Introductory Description*, New York: Russel Sage Foundation, 1922.

———. *The Long View: Papers and Addresses* (1930), Eds. J. C. Colcord and R.Z.S. Mann, Dubuque, IA: Brown, 1971.

Riemer, S., Urban personality reconsidered, *Community Structure and Analysis*, Ed. M. B. Sussman, New York: Crowell, 1959, 433-444.

Rittel, W. J., and Webber, M. M., Dilemmas in a general theory of planning, *Policy Sciences*, 4, June 1973, 155-169.

Roderick, T., Johnny can learn to negotiate, *Educational Leadership*, 45, December 1987/January 1988, 87-90.

Rogers, C. R., Dealing with psychological tensions, *Journal of Applied Behavioral Science*, 1, January/March 1965, 6-24.

————. The formative tendency, *Journal of Humanist Psychology*, 18, Winter 1978, 23-26.

Rosenberg, M., and Brody, R., *Systems Serving People: A Breakthrough in Service Delivery*, Cleveland: Case Western University, 1974.

Ross, M. G., and Lappin B., The role of the professional worker, *Community Organization* (1955), New York: Harper & Row, 1967, 203-231.

Rothman, J., Three models of community organization, *Strategies of Community Organization*, Eds. F. M. Cox, J. L. Erlich, J. Rothman, and J. E. Tropman. Itasca, IL: Peacock, 1970, 20-36.

————. The diffusion and adoption of innovations, *Planning and Organizing for Social Change*, New York: Columbia University Press, 1974, 417-483, 516-524.

Rouhana, N. N. and Kelman, H. C. (1994). Promoting joint thinking in international conflicts: A . . . continuing workshop. *Journal of Social Issues,* 50(1), 157-178.

Sanders, I. T., *The Community: An Introduction to a Social System* (1958), New York: Ronald Press, 1975.

Schoenberg, S. P., Criteria for the evaluation of neighborhood viability in working class and poor areas in core cities, *Social Problems*, 27, October 1979, 69-78.

Schon, D. A., *The Reflective Practitioner: How Professionals Think in Action*, New York: Basic Books, 1983.

Schwartz, W., The social worker in the group, *Social Welfare Forum: 1961*, New York: Columbia University Press, 146-171.

Seiler, J. A., *Systems Analysis in Organizational Behavior*, Homewood, IL: Dorsey/Irwin, 1967.

Shonholz, R., Neighborhood justice systems, *Mediation Quarterly*, 5, September 1984, 3-30.

Siporin, M., *An Introduction to Social Work Practice*, New York: Macmillan, 1975.

———. Practice theory and vested interest, *Social Service Review*, 52, September 1978, 418-436.

Skynner, A. C., Boundaries, *Social Work Today*, 5, August 1974, 290-294.

Staut, M., The social worker as an advocate in adult protective services, *Social Work*, 30, May/June 1985, 204-208.

Stein, I. L., Systems theory and social work, *Systems Theory, Science, and Social Work*, Metuchen, NJ: Scarecrow Press, 1974, 29-57.

Szent-Gyorgi, A., Science views the nuclear crisis, *Proceedings of the National Conference of Scientists on Survival*, New York City, June 15-17, 1962, Mimeographed.

Taylor, A. J. P., *The Second World War*, New York: G. P. Putnam, 1975.

Thyer, B. A., Contingency analysis: Towards a unified theory for social work practice, *Social Work*, 32, March/April 1987, 150-157.

Turner, F. J., Ed., *Social Work Treatment: Interlocking Theoretical Approaches* (1974), New York: Free Press, 1979.

Vickery, A., A systems approach to social work intervention: Its uses for work with individuals and families, *British Journal of Social Work*, 4, Winter 1974, 389-404.

Von Bertalanffy, L., The organism considered as a physical system (1940), *General System Theory*, New York: Braziller, 1968, 120-138.

———. *A Systems View of Man*, Ed. P. La Violette, Boulder, CO: Westview Press, 1981.

Vosler, N. R., A systems model for child protective services, *Journal of Social Work Education*, 25, Winter 1988, 20-28.

Wagley, C., and Harris, M., A typology of Latin American subcultures, *American Anthropologist*, 57, June 1955, 428-451.

Warfel, D. J., Maloney, D. M., and Blase, K. Consumer feedback in human service programs, *Social Work*, 26, March 1981, 151-156.

Warren, R. L., The conflict intersystem and the change agent, *Journal of Conflict Resolution*, 8, September 1964, 231-241.

————. and Hyman, H. H., Purposive community change in consensus and dissensus situations, *Community Mental Health Journal*, 2, Winter 1966, 293-300.

————. Types of purposive social change at the community level, *Readings in Community Organization Practice*, Eds. R. M. Kramer and H. Specht, Englewood Cliffs: Prentice-Hall, 1969, 205-222.

————. *Truth, Love and Social Change*, Chicago: Rand McNally, 1971.

————. *The Community in America* (1963), Chicago: Rand McNally, 1972.

Watson, M., *Proximics Behavior: A Cross-Cultural Study*, the Hague: Mouton, 1970.

Webber, M. M., Systems planning for social policy, *Readings in Community Organization Practice*, Eds. R. M. Kramer and H. Specht, Englewood Cliffs: Prentice-Hall, 1969, 417-424.

Weick, A., Reframing the person-in-environment perspective, *Social Work*, 26, March 1981, 140-143.

Weingarten, H., Strategic planning for divorce mediation, *Social Work*, 31, May/June 1986, 194-200.

————. and Leas, S., Levels of marital conflict model, *American Journal of Orthopsychiatry*, 57, July 1987, 407-417.

Whiteman, M., Fanshel, D., and Grundy, J. F., Cognitive-behavioral interventions aimed at anger of parents at risk of child abuse, *Social Work*, 32, November/December 1987, 469-474.

Woodger, J. H., *Biological Principles*, London: Kegan Paul, Trench, & Trubner, 1929.

Zimbalist, S. E., Community equilibrium: A case study in the curtailment of service, *Social Service Review*, 35, March 1961, 59-65.

Index

Page numbers followed by the letter "f" indicate figures; those followed by the letter "t" indicate tables.

Order Your Own Copy of
This Important Book for Your Personal Library!

SOCIAL WORK PRACTICE
A Systems Approach, Second Edition

_____ in hardbound at $39.95 (ISBN: 0-7890-0137-3)

_____ in softbound at $19.95 (ISBN: 0-7890-0246-9)

COST OF BOOKS_____

OUTSIDE USA/CANADA/
MEXICO: ADD 20%_____

POSTAGE & HANDLING_____
(US: $3.00 for first book & $1.25
for each additional book)
Outside US: $4.75 for first book
& $1.75 for each additional book)

SUBTOTAL_____

IN CANADA: ADD 7% GST_____

STATE TAX_____
(NY, OH & MN residents, please
add appropriate local sales tax)

FINAL TOTAL_____
(If paying in Canadian funds,
convert using the current
exchange rate. UNESCO
coupons welcome.)

☐ **BILL ME LATER:** ($5 service charge will be added)
(Bill-me option is good on US/Canada/Mexico orders only;
not good to jobbers, wholesalers, or subscription agencies.)

☐ Check here if billing address is different from
shipping address and attach purchase order and
billing address information.

Signature_____

☐ **PAYMENT ENCLOSED: $**_____

☐ **PLEASE CHARGE TO MY CREDIT CARD.**

☐ Visa   ☐ MasterCard   ☐ AmEx   ☐ Discover
☐ Diners Club
Account # _____

Exp. Date _____

Signature _____

Prices in US dollars and subject to change without notice.

NAME _____

INSTITUTION _____

ADDRESS _____

CITY _____

STATE/ZIP _____

COUNTRY _____ COUNTY (NY residents only) _____

TEL _____ FAX _____

E-MAIL_____
May we use your e-mail address for confirmations and other types of information? ☐ Yes   ☐ No

Order From Your Local Bookstore or Directly From
The Haworth Press, Inc.
10 Alice Street, Binghamton, New York 13904-1580 • USA
TELEPHONE: 1-800-HAWORTH (1-800-429-6784) / Outside US/Canada: (607) 722-5857
FAX: 1-800-895-0582 / Outside US/Canada: (607) 772-6362
E-mail: getinfo@haworth.com
PLEASE PHOTOCOPY THIS FORM FOR YOUR PERSONAL USE.

BOF96

OVERSEAS DISTRIBUTORS OF HAWORTH PUBLICATIONS

AUSTRALIA
Edumedia
Level 1, 575 Pacific Highway
St. Leonards, Australia 2065
(mail only) PO Box 1201
Crows Nest, Australia 2065
Tel: (61) 2 9901–4217 / Fax: (61) 2 9906-8465

CANADA
Haworth/Canada
450 Tapscott Road, Unit 1
Scarborough, Ontario M1B 5W1
Canada
(Mail correspondence and orders only. No returns or telephone inquiries. Canadian currency accepted.)

DENMARK, FINLAND, ICELAND, NORWAY & SWEDEN
Knud Pilegaard
Knud Pilegaard Marketing
Mindevej 45
DK-2860 Soborg, Denmark
Tel: (45) 396 92100

ENGLAND & UNITED KINGDOM
Alan Goodworth
Roundhouse Publishing Group
62 Victoria Road
Oxford OX2 7QD, U.K.
Tel: 44–1865–521682 / Fax: 44–1865-559594
E-mail: 100637.3571@CompuServe.com

GERMANY, AUSTRIA & SWITZERLAND
Bernd Feldmann
Heinrich Roller Strasse 21
D–10405 Berlin, Germany
Tel: (49) 304–434–1621 / Fax: (49) 304–434–1623
E-mail: BFeldmann@t-online.de

JAPAN
Mrs. Masako Kitamura
MK International, Ltd.
1–50–7–203 Itabashi
Itabashi–ku
Tokyo 173, Japan

KOREA
Se–Yung Jun
Information & Culture Korea
Suite 1016, Life Combi Bldg.
61–4 Yoido–dong
Seoul, 150–010, Korea

MEXICO, CENTRAL AMERICA & THE CARIBBEAN
Mr. L.D. Clepper, Jr.
PMRA: Publishers Marketing & Research Association
P.O. Box 720489
Jackson Heights, NY 11372 USA
Tel/Fax: (718) 803–3465
E-mail: clepper@usa.pipeline.com

NEW ZEALAND
Brick Row Publishing Company, Ltd.
Attn: Ozwald Kraus
P.O. Box 100–057
Auckland 10, New Zealand
Tel/Fax: (64) 09–410–6993

PAKISTAN
Tahir M. Lodhi
Al-Rehman Bldg., 2nd Fl.
P.O. Box 2458
65–The Mall
Lahore 54000, Pakistan
Tel/Fax: (92) 42–724–5007

PEOPLE'S REPUBLIC OF CHINA & HONG KONG
Mr. Thomas V. Cassidy
Cassidy and Associates
470 West 24th Street
New York, NY 10011 USA
Tel: (212) 727–8943 / Fax: (212) 727–8539

PHILIPPINES, GUAM & PACIFIC TRUST TERRITORIES
I.J. Sagun Enterprises, Inc.
Tony P. Sagun
2 Topaz Rd. Greenheights Village
Ortigas Ave. Extension Tatay, Rizal
Republic of the Philippines
P.O. Box 4322 (Mailing Address)
CPO Manila 1099
Tel/Fax: (63) 2–658–8466

SOUTH AMERICA
Mr. Julio Emöd
PMRA: Publishers Marketing & Research Assoc.
Rua Joauim Tavora 629
São Paulo, SP 04015001 Brazil
Tel: (55) 11 571–1122 / Fax: (55) 11 575-6876

SOUTHEAST ASIA & THE SOUTH PACIFIC, SOUTH ASIA, AFRICA & THE MIDDLE EAST
The Haworth Press, Inc.
Margaret Tatich, Sales Manager
10 Alice Street
Binghamton, NY 13904–1580 USA
Tel: (607) 722–5857 ext. 321 / Fax: (607) 722–3487
E-mail: getinfo@haworth.com

RUSSIA & EASTERN EUROPE
International Publishing Associates
Michael Gladishev
International Publishing Associates
c/o Mazhdunarodnaya Kniga
Bolshaya Yakimanka 39
Moscow 117049 Russia
Fax: (095) 251–3338
E-mail: russbook@online. ru

LATVIA, LITHUANIA & ESTONIA
Andrea Hedgecock
c/o Iki Tareikalavimo
Kaunas 2042
Lithuania
Tel/Fax: (370) 777-0241 / E-mail: andrea@soften.ktu.lt

SINGAPORE, TAIWAN, INDONESIA, THAILAND & MALAYSIA
Steven Goh
APAC Publishers
35 Tannery Rd.
#10–06, Tannery Block
Singapore, 1334
Tel: (65) 747–8662 / Fax: (65) 747–8916
E-mail: sgohapac@signet.com.sg